Where Do I Start?

A Nutritionist's Guide to Naturally Managing Insulin Resistance and Type 2 Diabetes

D1607614

Table of Contents

Hummus Dippers

Bell Peppers with Hummus

Peach & Almonds

Sun Butter Pumpkin Protein Balls

Roasted Turkey Breast & Carrots

House Salad

Steamed White Fish with Tomato & Olive Sauce

Steamed Asparagus

Zucchini Noodles with Salmon

Saffron Chicken Kebab with Salad

Steamed Green Beans

Turmeric Beef Stew

Spaghetti Squash Chow Mein

Week Two

Week Two Meal Plan

Detox Green Smoothie

Scrambled Eggs with Peppers & Kale

Creamy Blueberry Smoothie

Oatmeal with Raspberries

Spinach & Salsa Omelette

Simple Salmon Salad

Simple Lentil Flatbread

Creamy Carrot Soup

Turkey & Spinach Wrap

Chicken Tikka Salad

Herb & Garlic Quinoa

Grilled Shrimp Salad

Turmeric & Ginger Butternut Squash Stew

Sweet Potato Shepherd's Pie

Steamed Asparagus & Zucchini

Lemon Cilantro Cod with Peppers

Slow Cooker BBQ Pulled Pork

Pan Seared Chicken with Garlicky Cranberry Sauce

Carrots & Broccoli

Week Three

Week Three Meal Plan

Cinnamon Pear Oatmeal

Kiwi Lime Smoothie

Black Bean Egg White Omelette

Fluffy Kale & Mushroom Egg White Omelette

Asian Veggie Omelette

Slow Cooker Cod & Sea Veggie Soup

Sheet Pan Roasted Chicken & Veggies

Spicy Shrimp, Quinoa & Spinach

Salmon with Rice & Greens

Rosemary Lemon Chicken Skillet

Okra & Beef Stew

Brussels Sprouts Slaw with Chicken

Lemony Cod & Herbed Rice

Week Four

Week Four Meal Plan

- Cinnamon Protein Oats
- Berry Avocado Smoothie
- Blueberry Protein Smoothie
- Mushroom & Tofu Scramble
- Quinoa & Egg Breakfast Plate
- Pear & Kale Protein Smoothie
- Grain-Free Flax Bread
- Chicken, Asparagus & Sweet Potato
- Spinach & Sausage Egg Muffins
- Shrimp Zoodle Stir Fry
- Spicy Edamame Fried Cauliflower Rice
- Zucchini Noodles with Cauliflower Alfredo
- One Pan Steak Fajitas
- Seared Cod & Lemon White Beans
- Pressure Cooker Beef & Veggie Stew

Week Five

Week Five Meal Plan

- Oil-Free Scrambled Egg Whites
- Sweet Potato Hashbrowns
- Fruit & Egg Snack Plate
- Turkey Sausage Scramble
- Eggs n' Guac Breakfast Bowl
- Triple Berry Protein Bowl
- Asparagus & Mushroom Frittata

One Pot Poached Chicken with Broccoli & Sweet Potato

Broccoli & Mushroom Fried Rice

Coconut Chive Flatbread

Salmon Salad Lettuce Wraps

Tuna & Kale Chips

Sheet Pan Roasted Chicken & Veggies

Mayo-Dijon Salmon with Broccoli

Turkey & Vegetable Soup

One Pan Lemon Garlic Shrimp, Broccoli & Cauliflower Rice

Steamed Asparagus

Balsamic Dijon Chicken Thighs with Broccoli

Week Six

Week Six Meal Plan

Creamy Blueberry Smoothie

Chia Oats with Kiwi

Avocado Breakfast Toast

Cinnamon Oatmeal Pancakes

Fried Egg

Chocolate Strawberry Chia Pudding

Creamy Carrot Soup

Cobb Salad

Smoked Salmon Wrapped Avocado

Hummus & Veggies Snack Box

One Pan Chicken Fajita Bowls

Why I wrote this book

As a nutritionist, I work with people who have tried every diet and gimmick out there: cabbage soup diet, low fat, dirty keto, Weight Watchers, meal replacement drinks or bars, and more. I get it because I did the same thing. I spent years trying to lose weight and get healthy—I would lose a few pounds only to gain the weight back and start over. I hated my body and spent my most of my adult life on a "diet." That is no way to live! It was only when I began studying nutrition that I learned how to use real food to change my health and weight. Finally, freedom from diets! Real health without any effort, this is what I want for you.

My clients come to me with multiple health issues and need more than a six-week "lose ten pounds" diet. They need a complete lifestyle overhaul. They are tired of constant dieting and quick fixes that don't work. Together, we work to create a healthy life and diet that is sustainable, enjoyable, and easy to follow. But not every person has the option of working with a nutritionist.

People are busy and many do not have time to sit down and read a four-hundred-page book explaining how to create better health and deal with their specific health issue. My clients asked me if I could create an easy-to-read book that gave them the facts about their health issue and how to fix it. They didn't want to need a science or medical degree to understand the explanations, nor did they want to read endless pages of "fluff" before getting to the point. I listened to their concerns and desires and the result is a series of e-books on different health issues. I hope that this book helps you create the amazing healthy life you deserve.

Introduction

Getting a diagnosis of type 2 diabetes or insulin resistance can be very scary! Our first thought is usually, "But I don't want to be diabetic!" We have visions of needles, blindness, and debilitating illness for the rest of our lives, which can be terrifying. We wonder if it's too late, and what we need to do next. We vow to clean up our diets and exercise regularly. And, for a while, we manage to do this until we slide back into old habits. We start reaching for old foods, skip the gym, start feeling sick again, and start another diet. This cycle of starting and stopping goes on and on.

As a holistic nutritionist, women often tell me stories of their visit to the doctor who advised them they were pre-diabetic or had type 2 diabetes. Either the doctor would tell them their numbers weren't high enough for medication yet, or they would write out a prescription for medication to lower their blood glucose levels. Then they would hand them a pamphlet and say, "You should eat healthier, exercise, and lose weight. Stop eating so much sugar. If you have any questions just make another appointment," as they rush them out the door; leaving the patient wondering 'where do I start?' Now, I'm not trying to say anything negative about doctors because I know they are very busy people trying to do their best. They have huge patient loads and limited time for each appointment, they do not have the luxury of spending hours working with each patient.

The doctor's advice is correct; diet, exercise, and even medication is all part of the solution. But knowing where to start and understanding that the two keys to naturally managing type 2 diabetes are changing your diet and lifestyle and creating healthy new habits that will last a lifetime is the difference between success and failure. If you get your blood glucose under control and then go back to your old eating and exercise habits, you will get it back again, therefore the changes you make must be permanent.

This book is not a quick-fix diet to lose weight and fix your blood glucose levels, only for you to put the weight back on and have high numbers again when you stop your new healthy eating lifestyle, but a long-term plan that explains how to change your diet and lifestyle to manage your diabetes and obtain optimal health and energy for the rest of your life.

You will learn:

- What to eat
- The most important food to add to your diet for overall health
- Which exercise programs work best
- How to improve sleep
- How to remove toxins to allow your body to heal
- How to better deal with stress and balance your hormones.

I will provide you a step-by-step guide to implement these changes into your diet to remove added sugar and add in the healthy habits that will change your life for the better. I will also give you tips for working shiftwork, travelling, and provide a list of foods to avoid and supplements you may wish to consider. Also included is a six-week menu plan to transition you from the Standard American Diet to a healthy diet, with delicious recipes and tips.

There is a preconceived notion that type 2 diabetes is "your fault" because of a lack of exercise and poor food choice, but this isn't the full story. In this book you will come to understand why calories are not all the same and why the food choices you make now have a huge impact on your health for years to come. We will also look at how changing the type of food you eat has the biggest impact.

The rise in type 2 diabetes is a complex social issue related to food choices, exercise, exposure to advertisements, access to public health, access to support for health-related issues, income, toxins, obesogens, pesticides, endocrine disruptors, and food product manipulation. Some doctors will tell you type 2 diabetes is a disease with a natural progression, and there is nothing you can do to prevent the inevitable end of blindness or early death. This is not true! Studies have shown a change in lifestyle, including the foods we eat, can and will manage your type 2 diabetes symptoms. Don't give up! There is hope! I have witnessed amazing transformations with a change in diet and lifestyle.

Type 2 diabetes doesn't only impact blood glucose levels, but our heart health, immunity, digestive health, blood pressure, and cholesterol. We need to address all these issues at the same time. There are many great dietary plans out there, but each only addresses one issue, which I believe is a flaw. There is no diet that works for every person because we are all unique and need to be able to create a plan that works for us as individuals.

We all need a starting point of knowledge that will help us create our new healthy lifestyle. This book will provide basic nutritional information that will help to reduce sodium intake, improve heart health, reduce cholesterol levels, boost nutrition, immune health, and improve digestive health. I will explain both low glycemic and ketogenic diets that can be used to lower blood glucose, as well as using intermittent fasting to improve cell response and increase weight loss. By following this guide, you will receive the best plan for lowering your glucose levels, improving your overall health, and learning how to permanently change your habits to create a healthy lifestyle forever.

I believe we have the power to make incredible changes in our life if we are given the information we need in a style both simple to understand and implement. Therefore, I have tried to avoid using technical terms and did my best to make complicated issues easy to understand. Most people who buy a book never read past the first chapter, perhaps because of the length or maybe because many books are filled with technical jargon that make it confusing and overwhelming to read. For this reason, I have kept this book shorter and more to-the-point while still giving you all the knowledge you need to make the necessary changes for better health.

The information contained in this book will guide you in making the best choices for you and your family and the decisions you make will have a powerful impact on your overall health. You will also need to decide which changes you can, or are willing, to make. Only you can make a difference in your health and life. Only you can manage your diagnosis of type 2 diabetes. I can give you all the information, tips, and encouragement you need, but at the end of the day, only you can make the necessary changes in your diet and lifestyle. If you are reading this book; then I know that you are ready to make a change for the better. I believe in you. You can choose to make changes gradually or all at once, depending on your comfort level. I encourage you to discuss your new diet and lifestyle changes with your doctor and be sure to have your glucose levels checked regularly to track your progress.

In this book I will refer to the general term of "type 2 diabetes" rather than continually writing out "insulin resistance / type 2 diabetes" but the information provided works for both.

If you are reading this book to help a child, please note that children should never be put on a calorie-restricted diet without discussing it first with their pediatrician, as they require a specific caloric intake to continue growing. Changing their current diet to a healthier version can be done in conjunction with or without caloric restriction. With kids, it is much easier to make gradual changes so there is less resistance and risk of creating food-related disorders, such as bulimia or anorexia, in the future.

Any changes made should be for the entire family so as not to single-out one member. After all, you want your entire family to be healthier, not just one person. Never forbid any specific food but have all things in moderation. If you fill your fridge and cupboards with healthy options and the occasional unhealthy choice, your overall health will still improve. Just as with adults, if you tell a child they can never have a specific food item again, they will crave it, and may hide these foods or binge eat them when available. Teach your children that life is about balance in all things—

teach them to have a better relationship with food, and that food is for nourishment, not comfort.

If you are making changes in your home for a child that has prediabetes or type 2 diabetes, information specific to them can be found in later chapters. However, I still recommend reading the entire book so you gain knowledge about carbohydrates, proteins, fats, foods to avoid, and exercise that can help the whole family. Be sure to work alongside their pediatrician, as their needs may change as they grow.

Always check with your physician to ensure that any new dietary program will work with your specific needs and talk to your doctor before adding any supplements or starting a new exercise program.

Congratulations on making the decision to live a healthier, happier life! Now, let's get started.

Type 2 Diabetes - What Is It?

Type 2 diabetes, or diabetes mellitus, is a problem in the way the body either produces or uses insulin. It is also sometimes called non-insulin dependent diabetes or adult-onset diabetes. However, with the dramatic rise in the number of children with type 2 diabetes, the term "adult diabetes" is rarely used anymore.

Insulin is a hormone produced in the pancreas and is required for carbohydrate, fat, and protein to be metabolized (broken down, absorbed, and used) in the body. To put it simply, all carbohydrates break down into glucose. The pancreas produces insulin, which allows the glucose to enter our cells for energy. If we consume a diet that has too many carbohydrates over a long period of time, we may develop type 2 diabetes because our cells no longer recognize the insulin (insulin resistance), and therefore our pancreas must produce more to try to give our cells the energy we require. The pancreas may "burn out" and become unable to keep up with the additional required insulin production, therefore leaving too much blood glucose in our system (hyperglycemia), while leaving our cells starved for energy.

Fat has little, if any, effect on blood glucose levels, although a high fat intake does appear to contribute to insulin resistance. Protein has a minimal effect on blood glucose levels if we have adequate insulin in our body. However, with insulin deficiency, gluconeogenesis (the creation of glucose from non-carbohydrate sources such as protein) quickly contributes to an elevated blood glucose level.

Before the development of type 2 diabetes, people were frequently diagnosed with prediabetes (also called "impaired glucose tolerance"), which is categorized by higher-than-normal blood sugar levels (fasting glucose of 100–125 mg/dl in the U.S. or 6.1mmol/L to 6.9 mmol/L in Canada) and is the first step in insulin resistance. There are approximately fifty-eight million Americans with prediabetes, many of whom are unaware of their illness.

Prediabetes can be blamed on a diet of refined carbohydrates, saturated fat, excessive caloric intake, lack of exercise, industrial pollutants, increased inflammatory markers, hormonal imbalances, inadequate sleep, and nutrient deficiencies. Research shows that due to the destructive nature of high levels of insulin, prediabetes is usually accompanied by high cholesterol, high blood pressure, heart disease, non-alcoholic fatty liver disease, and obesity, therefore it is imperative to lower insulin levels in order to address the other accompanying illnesses.

Insulin resistance is the next stage, occurring when the body doesn't use or recognize insulin properly. It may be part of metabolic syndrome (a grouping of risk factors including excess belly fat, high blood pressure, and high blood sugar levels) which increases risk of diabetes, heart disease, and stroke, and is found in approximately 40% of Americans. Insulin resistance is usually associated with obesity (especially around the middle), fatigue after eating, sugar cravings (especially during menstruation), high triglycerides and blood pressure, poor cholesterol, and chronic inflammation. Individuals with metabolic syndrome also report poorer health-related quality of life physically, mentally, and emotionally.

Obesity is a major risk factor for type 2 diabetes because when our fat cells (adipocytes) are full, they secrete several biological molecules (such as resistin, leptin, tumor necrosis factor, and cortisol) that slow the effect of insulin, impair the use of glucose in the skeletal muscles, promote glucose production in the liver, and impair the release of insulin by the pancreas. The greater the number of fat cells we have, the less we secrete compounds that promote insulin use (adiponectin). In this way, excess fat is associated with insulin resistance. In the beginning, blood glucose levels may remain level despite the insulin resistance as the pancreas compensates by producing more insulin. As metabolic stress increases, the pancreas can no longer keep up, and insulin resistance becomes evident. As the disease progresses, the pancreas burns out and begins to produce less and less insulin, and full-blown diabetes takes hold.

There are other risk factors for type 2 diabetes, including a family history of diabetes, age (over 45s), race/ethnicity (such as Native American, African American, Hispanic American, Native Australian, and Asian American), those with hypertension, high triglycerides, and women with polycystic ovary syndrome. Now, this doesn't mean if you fall into one of these categories you are guaranteed to get type 2 diabetes, only that these groups have a higher risk of getting it.

According to the World Health Organization, diabetes is the leading cause of blindness, kidney failure, heart attacks, strokes, and lower limb amputation. And, according to the Centre for Disease Control, thirty-four million adults have diabetes, and eighty-eight million adults have prediabetes. Childhood type 2 diabetes is rising at a rate of approximately 5% every year, similar to the rates of childhood obesity. These are scary statistics that are increasing every year.

Our bodies are an integrated, interdependent unit that is in a delicate balance, and it is no wonder that, as we develop prediabetes, we often develop high cholesterol, non-alcoholic fatty liver disease, and digestive disorders. Because every cell of our body needs glucose, diabetes affects every cell and organ in our body and therefore people with diabetes are at a greater risk of heart disease, stroke, high blood pressure, cancer, blindness, and atherosclerosis.

So how do we know if we are becoming prediabetic or have insulin resistance? A simple test your doctor can do is a fasting insulin test. This test measures the insulin levels that are in your blood when they are not impacted by food, detecting insulin resistance long before a fasting blood glucose test does. This test shows the early signs of metabolic dysfunction before a person becomes diabetic. Catching this early allows for better intervention with diet, exercise, and lifestyle. Sadly, many doctors do not order a fasting insulin test but rely on the fasting glucose test. They are trained to measure fasting blood glucose levels and are not normally concerned until your blood sugar levels reach 110 mg/dL. Once you reach this level, doctors advise you to change your diet and lifestyle, but you may be (and probably are) already insulin resistant and on your way to becoming a type 2 diabetic.

Let's say your fasting blood glucose is at 80 mg/dL, and you have high fasting insulin of 20 mg/dL. This means your pancreas has to pump out extra insulin to keep your blood glucose level stable and within the "desirable" range. Measuring insulin is the critical piece in determining a person's risk for diabetes. If you obtain a fasting insulin test, please note that the average range is normally too high for the average person. I prefer to work with an optimal range, which metabolic health experts agree is a much narrower range of 3 to 5 mIU/mL. If your numbers are higher than ten, you are beginning to develop a problem you need to address, and if your level is over fifteen, your levels are significantly elevated, and you must address this immediately. Compare this to the "normal range" used by many doctors, in which anything less than 25 mIU/mL is considered normal. Using a narrower range can make a big difference to your health and allow you to detect problems earlier.

Multiple scientific studies have shown a diet high in refined carbohydrates plays a major role in the cause, prevention, and treatment of type 2 diabetes. Our modern diet is heavily influenced by carbohydrates. We have either toast, cereal, a bagel, or breakfast sandwiches for our first meal of the day, often with a cup of coffee with cream and sugar. Then, our midmorning snack might be a doughnut at the morning office meeting, or a muffin from a coffee shop. Lunch is a sandwich, or a hamburger with a white bun, pasta, or perhaps a microwavable processed frozen meal. Afternoon snack is cookies, a muffin, or some other quick snack from the vending machine, washed down with more caffeine. Dinner will be protein of some sort, vegetables and a dinner roll or slice of bread. This is all packed into a very busy day while we are trying to keep our family fed on a budget and get through the day until we finally collapse into bed exhausted only to do it all over again tomorrow. Did I miss anything?

I believe people try to eat healthily and trust food labels on the side of the boxes and packages indicating "added vitamins" or "a full serving of vegetables" or "part of a complete breakfast." I see women looking at labels in the grocery store to determine what they are buying, and I hear them talking about the rising cost of groceries and inflation. The fact is that processed foods are cheaper and last longer on the shelf, and the more processed the food, the cheaper it is. When we are trying to feed a family on a limited budget, this has a huge impact. The problem with this is the massive amount of processed carbohydrates we eat is killing us. Processed carbohydrates do not have the same nutrition, nor do they contain the fibre necessary, to slow our digestion and therefore glucose absorption. And while the low cost may be helpful now, we will pay a huge price in the long term. We need to get over our addiction to processed carbohydrates and change our diets for the better.

Lifestyle changes can result in managing (or putting it in remission) pre-diabetes and type 2 diabetes. Weight loss, exercising, and healthy eating habits are key for preventing progression into type 2 diabetes (insulin dependent), and the increased health risks that come with it.

In this plan, we will:

- Incorporate more natural healthy foods.
- Remove all artificial sweeteners (which trick the body into thinking there is glucose, therefore increasing insulin).

- Reduce inflammation by removing processed carbohydrates and refined poor quality oils.
- Increase intake of fibre rich foods which feed our gut bacteria and boost immunity.
- Lower cholesterol.
- Allow for better nutrient absorption.
- Ensure proper elimination (to remove toxins, waste, and excess hormones), address nutrient deficiencies, reduce stress, and add in proper exercise.

But I am going to be honest with you, this is easier said than done. We are a generation of processed carb addicts. If weight loss was easy, no one would need to diet. If healthy eating and creating a healthy lifestyle were easy, no one would need to work with a nutritionist like myself. It is estimated that forty-five million people a year go on a diet, and they are spending thirty-three billion dollars on weight loss products. That is a staggering number! And sadly, most weight loss products and traditional diets don't work. They may lose weight but will regain it (and sometimes more) within a year. There are so many different diets on the market, with more and more created each year. Atkins, Weight Watchers, low fat, low carb, keto, the Mediterranean, paleo, and so on. How do we choose and how can we make this easier, cheaper, and provide better results?

The answer is by creating a healthy lifestyle that is sustainable, balanced, easy-to-follow, and works for you. We need to create better habits, so healthy living doesn't require thought or effort. We need to get back to basics of eating real, unprocessed, unaltered food the way Mother Nature intended. We need to make finding healthy food on road trips as easy as the processed packaged crap we find on the shelves in gas stations. We need to make "fast food" mean eating an apple on the run, not a highly caloric hamburger, fries, and soda. We need to ensure the next generation of children is healthier than us, not sicker. And you need to create a lifestyle that works for you and your family so you can stick to it long-term. If you are a person that likes to eat meat, suddenly becoming a vegan will not work. If your work dictates eating in restaurants most of the time, then a home-cooked approach isn't going to work for you. This plan will provide different options so you can implement what will work for your own lifestyle.

You may already know some of what I am going to tell you, but are you doing it? Alternatively, some of what I'm going to tell you might be new, and you might even be thinking, "Oh, that's easy for her to say, but I can't because...." So I am asking you to keep an open mind. We all have excuses as to why we can't do things, but if we absolutely have to, we find a way. If you were told tomorrow that if you ate processed sugar you would die, would you eat it or would you stop eating it? Of course, you would cut it out of your life because you knew that your life depended on it. The problem is that our life *does* depend on it, but the results are so slow and insidious that we don't realize the damage we are doing to our body. It's like a piece of metal that is slowly rusting, but it takes so long to happen we don't see it until it is an issue.

We are going to be making changes in our diet, exercise, and lifestyle. I am going to give you some tips you can choose to implement right away to start making positive changes and get results quickly. I am going to ask you to change old habits and make some difficult life decisions. Be honest with yourself about the choices you are currently making and the ones you need to change. Your immediate response might be that you cannot make a change because of such and such. But is it the truth, or an excuse made for convenience?

I worked with a client who was addicted to Coca-Cola, drank a 4-litre bottle of it every day and took microwave meals to work daily because they were cheap and filling. Her blood glucose numbers were off the chart, she suffered from non-alcoholic fatty liver disease, obesity, and high blood pressure. She insisted that she could not eat healthy because she could not afford it. In her mind, healthy vegetables were expensive and not within her budget.

When I had her track where she spent her money and what she was buying, we found that she was spending over twenty percent of her food budget on pop, chips, cookies, breakfast cereals, and instant microwave food for her lunch at work. When she stopped buying these items and replaced them with water (from the tap), fruit such as apples and oranges, oatmeal, and eggs for breakfast, and started preparing her lunch at home, she found that not only could she buy healthy food, but she had money left over.

We all have habits of convenience and often feel it's the only option because we have done it that way for years. But when we take a step back and take look at a situation with a different lens, we may come up with a better solution. I'm going to ask you to take a look at your current habits to determine which are helping and which are hurting you and what changes you are willing to make. Don't be afraid to ask someone for help or advice on your specific situation in order to get some ideas on how to make positive changes. A fresh perspective often yields new ideas.

Mindset Matters

Changing our habits is one of the keys to managing type 2 diabetes and creating a healthy balanced life, but it is impossible to change our habits without the right mindset. Mindset is a pattern of thinking and the starting place for a new healthy life. For example, if you are a happy positive person, then you probably tend to have a positive mindset. When things go wrong (because life is like that) you react to problems in a different manner than a person whose mindset is negative. A person with a negative mindset tends to be an "all or nothing" person. They believe things "always" go wrong and do not see the positive aspects of their life.

If you approach managing your type 2 diabetes with the attitude of "I *should* eat healthy" or "I *might* change my habits" then I am telling you right now, you will fail. Not to be harsh, but you need to change your mindset to "*I am*" and keep reminding yourself of this new attitude. Telling yourself that you should eat healthy is a big difference from *I am eating healthy*. One is a wishy-washy maybe, while the other is a declaration.

When we want to change our diet and lifestyle, we need to adopt a new mindset, that of a healthy person. Instead of thinking "I am a person on a diet," you need to think of yourself as a healthy person living a healthy lifestyle. Whenever you look in the mirror or at your reflection in a window, I want you to say (in your mind or out loud) *I am a healthy person*. And when you walk into a kitchen or restaurant, tell yourself again, *I am a healthy person*. Put a sign on your refrigerator so it is visible when you feel like having a snack, use it as your computer screensaver at work, put reminders on your phone, and sticky notes on your car's dashboard.

Tell yourself *I am a healthy person* throughout the day for thirty days and see the power of your words. We believe what we hear repeatedly. Don't believe me? I once had a friend who was told by her mother that she was stupid and would never learn to read. As a result, my friend believed her mother and could not read. One day, she was at my house and told my mom that she was stupid and would never learn to read. My mom was furious (not at her, of course), and told her there were no stupid children, just people who needed a new way of thinking. Mom told her to tell herself *I am learning to read* every day while she practiced her reading. She began to work with my friend, and within two weeks she had taught her to read. As an adult, my friend has read hundreds of books and has a love of reading she has passed on to her own children. Imagine if she had never changed the message she was telling herself?

We create our own reality based on our thoughts, feelings, and emotions, which determine our actions and reactions. What we believe and feel impacts our actions. If you are not committed to your new lifestyle, then your feeling of uncertainty will impact your actions. While nutrition is important, mindset is equally as important. If you tell yourself you are a healthy person and make the decision to live as a healthy person, then your actions will reflect your belief. You will make better food choices, you will exercise because that is what a healthy person does, and you will have a better life balance overall because that is what a healthy person has. What you think impacts how you feel and how you feel dictates how you act.

A diet mentality is a narrow short-term focus that most people fall into. I know I was a constant dieter for many years and fell prey to all the marketing schemes promising instant results. Restrictive diets mess up our metabolisms and can make us heavier and unhealthier than previously, can impact our mental and emotional health, and can create the idea that we are destined to be overweight. To manage type 2 diabetes, we need to ditch the diet mentality and make way for a healthier approach that lasts forever.

Some examples of a diet mentality are:

❖ when we create rules around food, allowing ourselves to eat only certain foods in specific amounts. The cabbage-soup diet comes to mind.

❖ eliminating whole food groups (especially those that provide nutrition), such as all fruit.

❖ thinking food is either good or bad and associating your self-worth in relation to these foods. For example, "I am bad because I ate a donut."

❖ mainly prioritizing a specific number on a scale or body-fat percentage rather than better health and wellbeing.

❖ spending your money on pills, teas, creams, powders, or meal replacement products for fat loss rather than focusing on nutrition and health.

The diet mindset leads to guilt, frustration, anxiety, and poor self-worth. It also means you ignore listening to your body in favour of following strict, self-inflicted rules about what and when to eat. Feeling you have to "fix" your body in order to be happy and focusing on quick fixes (the latest diet pills or fad diet) to address "problem" areas. We look in the mirror and grab hold of our belly fat or thigh fat and feel we are not beautiful as long as we have the ability to hold fat in our fingers. We suck in our tummy and imagine how happy we will be when it's flat. We are always looking for the next way to "fix" our perceived flaws. In the end, a negative mindset will lead to failure.

Scientific studies and psychologists have indicated that how we see ourselves will determine our actions. If we think of ourselves as unhealthy or unworthy, we will act accordingly and avoid exercise and healthy eating. If we think of ourselves as a healthy person who is worthy of a healthy body, we will focus on positive outcomes such as having more energy, a longer life, better sleep, more strength, ability to prevent disease and illness, and a greater enjoyment of everyday living. By creating a healthy person mindset, you will manage your type 2 diabetes forever. Remember that healthy living is a journey, not a destination, so even if you are not as healthy as you want to be, you are still a healthy person who is getting healthier every day.

 The first step in a mindset change is to get real on your reason *why* you want to change your diet and lifestyle. One exercise I have found particularly useful with my clients is asking them why they want to manage their type 2 diabetes over and over until we get to the real, deep-down reason that will provide them with sustained motivation for change. These reasons are usually related to feelings of self-worth, a desire for a family, or being there long-term for family members.

Now you might be thinking that you are going to skip past this step, but I want you to take the time right now to complete this exercise. You may want to ask a friend or family member to help you or complete it in private if you prefer. This may bring up feelings or memories, so take the time you need to complete this exercise. Allow yourself to feel what you are feeling, accept it, and know that you are making these changes to be a healthier, happier person.

The next thing I am asking you to do is to set two short-term goals that are action-oriented, specific, and realistic. Setting a clear and specific goal, will allow you to track and measure your progress, and set yourself up for success. If you have a vague goal of "I want to lose weight" and you lose one pound, technically you have achieved your goal, but are you happy? If you have a vague goal of "I want to be healthier," what does this mean specially? Reducing your fasting insulin numbers? Being able to climb a set of stairs without feeling winded? Reducing your cholesterol numbers?

I am asking you to set realistic goals because if we set a goal that is never going to happen, we get frustrated and may quit working toward it. For example, if you set a goal to lose fifty pounds in a month, that is an unrealistic (and unhealthy) goal that you will not achieve. But if you set a goal to lose fifty pounds in six months, it would be more realistic. I want you to set yourself up for success.

A goal needs to be something we are motivated to work toward, something that excites us. Short-term goals can be more effective than only focusing on the end goal, especially if that end goal may take months to achieve. Try setting and achieving small goals such as drinking six glasses of water per day, eating fruit each day, or having a salad per day. When we achieve small goals, it provides the motivation to achieve another and another and before you know it you are hitting the big goals.

Track your progress using a calendar or journal so you can see your positive results. I like hanging a calendar on the wall and putting up a happy face sticker each day I achieve my goal. It is a physical reminder with an emotional cue. When you have achieved your short-term goal, give yourself a reward (but not with food), such as a new book, new workout shoes, a day to sleep in, a massage, or anything else that makes you feel good. Then, I want you to set two more goals. Continually setting and achieving small, short-term goals is key to staying on-track and creating healthy habits. Do not use food as a reward as we need to change from seeing food as a reward or punishment to that of providing nourishment for our body, as you are going to learn in this book.

Journaling is a great way to help stay focused on our goals, track our progress, and gives us a place to explore ideas, fears, and joy. At the end of each day, write about what went well in your journal. I know it's human nature to think about what went wrong, but remember, our thoughts dictate our actions and if we are thinking about something negative, it will not inspire us, and we will not have the same reaction. Focus on how you felt that day. What did you achieve? What went right? For example, have you eliminated or reduced your bloating or gas? Can you walk up the stairs without feeling out of breath? Did you walk away from the home-baked cookies in the lunch-room?

Focus more on the journey rather than the final goal on the scale. Celebrate each success! Remember, you are a person living a healthy lifestyle, not a person on a diet.

One complaint I hear over and over is that we don't want to give up our favourite foods. Well, guess what? You are not dieting—you are a person living a healthy lifestyle. You can still have those unhealthy foods, just choose to have them on a more limited basis, in smaller portions, and not as often. You may want to choose one meal a month that includes one of your favourite not-so-healthy foods. This is not a "cheat" meal because you are not dieting. This is your healthy lifestyle. Remember, healthy living is not all or nothing. Be realistic, even healthy people make unhealthy choices once in a while. The trick is to make sure that "once in a while" doesn't occur more than once a month. If that favourite food is high in sugar, you will also need to adjust your eating and activities to accommodate it.

Focus on what you *can* eat, not what you can't. I want you to write down all the different fruits, vegetables, berries, protein sources, and healthy grains that you *can* have—you will be amazed by how long the list is! Challenge yourself to try a new type of fruit or vegetable and expand your food choices. Try a new cultural food or way of cooking.

Ditch the guilt and body-shaming. If we think of food as a reward for good behavior and exercise as a punishment for bad behavior, then we will never have the mindset of a healthy person. Eating nutritious food is about self-love and self-worth. Exercise is about self-love and self-worth. You are worthy of a healthy, energetic strong body, and focusing on self-love and self-worth is a more powerful motivator than self-loathing. If you do catch yourself using negative self-talk, stop and change the message to something positive. If you catch yourself pinching a roll of fat in the mirror, stop and look yourself in the eyes and tell yourself, "I love you. You are worthy." If you joke about being the "fat friend," then stop right now. You are *not* your weight. Let me repeat that. You are not your weight. You are not the "fat friend" or "fat sister" and your weight is not a judgement of your self-worth. It is a number on the scale, at this moment in time, and can change. Your intelligence, kindness, positivity, creativity, and work ethic do not change, and they are the real reflection of the person you truly are.

Physical activity

Part of changing our mindset is choosing physical activities you love. If you hate a specific exercise, then telling yourself you will do it five times a week is not productive. Personally, I hate running but I like walking. If I set a goal to run five days per week, I would not do it because I would hate every minute of it. I would procrastinate and find every excuse under the sun to avoid it. But, if I set a goal to walk five days a week, I would achieve that goal because it is an activity I enjoy.

Incorporate different activities that will keep it interesting and avoid boredom. Try a new activity to see if the new healthy version of yourself likes it. You might find an activity you never thought you would be interested in. When my daughter was a teenager, she hated physical education class in school and group sports such as baseball, basketball, and soccer, but discovered a love of fencing. She went on to win a fencing competition in her age group and still loves the sport to this day.

Choose whether you want to participate in group activities, classes and events, or exercise alone. Perhaps you want a bit of both? Exercising in a group or even in a gym has been shown to be a great motivator. I always work out a bit harder when I am in the gym than when I am home alone. Be cautious of choosing activities that also include eating and drinking (for example, a team sport in which everyone goes for beer afterwards).

There's a famous quote from Jim Rohn that says we are the average of the five people we hang out with most. And for the most part, I think he is correct. If you hang out with people who take care of their health, are motivated, positive, and like to exercise, you are more likely to do the same. If you hang out with people who like to sit around and eat chips while watching television, then you are more likely to follow suit. It's okay to make new friends and try new activities, this doesn't mean you are abandoning your old friends but do expect a bit of resistance from them. Some will be very supportive of your new life, while others will feel threatened. Stand your ground and stick with your new healthy lifestyle. When they see how happy it makes you feel, they might feel inspired to join you.

When you find an activity you enjoy, make a commitment so that you don't revert to old habits. If you hire a trainer, schedule the appointments in advance so you can't skip them. Pay for the baseball jersey and tell your teammates they can count on you to be there. Book the babysitter so you can get to the gym. Making a monetary and verbal commitment sets your intention, and you are more likely to follow through.

And do not hide away until you reach a specific weight or size before participating in sports or going to the gym. I often hear people voice fears about going to the gym and exercising because they are embarrassed and think everyone will be looking at them. Not to burst your bubble, but most people are way too self-centered to be looking at you. They are focused on themselves, their music, or the television in front of them.

I once had a woman working out in front of me at the gym, and I guess she thought I was looking at her and bravely came up to talk to me about it. Honestly, she had to touch me on the arm before I even noticed she was there. I had my headphones in and was working through a problem in my head, so I never even noticed her other than she was on the machine I wanted next. I apologized for staring but then explained I didn't actually notice her other than to see how long she had left so I could work that machine into my circuit. She was embarrassed, and so was I, but we had a good laugh about it. And remember, everyone starts as a beginner, so never feel embarrassed about asking for help. Most gyms have staff members who will provide tours or give tips on how to use machines safely.

Mindful eating

In addition to changing the way we feel about exercise, I want you to make a change in the way you feel about food. Over the years, the concept of food has changed from providing nutrition, health, and longevity, and nourishing our body, to an idea that food is there to provide comfort, or to be used as a punishment or reward.

Throughout history, food has always been part of our culture and our celebrations of major life milestones such as marriage, the birth of a child, or a funeral. It is only within the last fifty years that food has become linked to human emotion. We turn to food when we are lonely, stressed, anxious, bored, sad, or feeling empty inside. Children are given sugary foods as a treat after the dentist or for a good report card or are sent to bed without supper for misbehaving. We mindlessly eat while watching television, not because we are hungry but because we are bored, because of television advertising, or old habits. We get stressed out at work and reach for the bag of cookies hidden in our desk drawer. Or maybe we have a fight with our spouse and reach for a piece of cake to make ourselves feel better. Over the last fifty years, humans have become more and more addicted to sugar and because sugar affects the dopamine in our brains (which give us a good feeling when we are sad, angry, or anxious), we reach for it constantly.

To create new habits, we are going to practice mindful and intuitive eating, which is a great way of stopping sugar addiction, listening to our body, breaking emotional eating habits, and changing our thoughts to those of a healthy person.

Mindful eating is about paying attention to the aroma, texture, taste, and flavour of a food, which teaches us to slow down and be more conscious about what we are eating. To do this, I want you to create an environment for eating that is peaceful and inviting. We all know eating on the run isn't good for our digestion, but did you know the atmosphere you create can also impact digestive health? Put away all distractions such as cell phones and turn off the television. Don't sit at your work desk or in front of a computer. Sit at a table and really focus on what you are eating. Enjoy the smell, the texture, the taste, and the feeling of enjoyment from your delicious and nutritious food. Put down your fork between bites. Take the time to eat slowly, chew thoroughly and savour every bite. Too often we eat quickly so we can dash off to do something else. Our lives have become so busy that we don't even taste our food anymore.

The Japanese have an expression, *hara hachi bu*, which means to eat until you are 80% full or no longer hungry. I think we can learn something from this, as our culture embraces the "eat until we are full" mentality, causing overeating, indigestion, bloating, and lethargy. By eating more slowly we will learn to notice when we have had enough food rather than just quickly eating everything on our plate. Research has shown that creating mindful eating habits can reduce emotional eating, binge eating, and improve digestive health.

If you are at home, have all the members of your family come to the table (without any distractions) and share the experiences of your day, talk about current events or any other positive topic that works for you. Learn to connect with your loved ones again. If you are at work, go to the lunchroom and eat while talking to coworkers instead of eating at your desk. If you are alone, try putting on some peaceful music and take your time to enjoy your meal. Slow down and let food nourish your body as it was meant to.

Intuitive eating is about trusting your body to know when it is hungry, learning that a food is not "bad" or "good," respecting your body, and treating yourself with kindness. Your body knows when you are hungry, but we often force ourselves to eat at scheduled times out of habit rather than hunger.

When my daughter was in school, I would nag at her to eat breakfast when she first woke up because I didn't want her to be hungry later and buy something unhealthy from a vending machine. She repeatedly told me that she wasn't hungry first thing in the morning, but I wouldn't listen. This caused a lot of arguments in the household until we came to a compromise. She would take something to school to eat for breakfast and eat when she was hungry. I was happy because I knew she was eating something healthy and not going hungry. She was happy because she could eat when she was truly hungry (and because I stopped nagging at her). Children are great at intuitive eating. Toddlers will stop eating when full and turn away from food or cry if the parent tries to make them eat more.

If you are eating when you are not hungry, ask yourself if you are you eating because of an old habit, or because you are stressed/bored/anxious/tired. Old habits can be hard to break. If, for example, you always have chips and beer when watching a movie, ask yourself what you can eat instead. If you are eating to fill a void, what else can you do instead of eating? Can you call a friend? Go for a walk? Exercise? Learn to listen to your body and know when you are truly hungry or thirsty rather than filling an emotional void, or because of old habits. Trust yourself to know when you are hungry and then to eat accordingly.

I am an evening snacker, and often eat because another person is eating even though I am not hungry. I realized that as a child if I didn't eat the snack foods when everyone else did, then there were none left for me to have later. This made me feel sad and left out, so I ate to avoid this feeling. Even now as an adult with my own home, I still find myself repeating the same behavior. Learning to understand our behaviors and triggers can be very helpful.

One way to break old habits is by putting a note on the fridge door to ask yourself *what you are feeling*—hungry or bored? If you know you will be tempted during an event (such as a movie night or when watching football), plan ahead and decide what you will do. Will you have healthier options available to eat? Will you stick to drinking herbal tea? Or will you change the event so old eating habits are not triggered?

Writing in your journal can help to track your emotions and learn the triggers that activate old habits, so you can address these and change your reactions. Creating a healthy lifestyle and new habits means we have to unlearn old habits and create new ones. This takes time and effort, but it is the difference between success and failure.

Let's talk cravings. We all have them but what do we do when a craving hits? When I have a food craving, one trick I use is "I can have it tomorrow if I still want it." If I am craving pie, for example, I tell myself that I can have it tomorrow. Most of the time I have forgotten the craving within an hour and no longer want the unhealthy food. If I still want the pie the next day, then I have a small portion of the best pie I can buy. I don't buy or make a full pie because I know I will eat too much of it (I love pie), so one piece is the perfect solution for me. I will sit quietly with my pie and slowly enjoy every bite without guilt.

Knowledge can be a powerful tool in changing our mindset. Knowing how a specific food helps our body can be a great way of reinforcing our new mindset of a healthy person. Learning about the nutritional value of different foods and what they provide our body can be a great motivator. Learn about different herbs and spices and the amazing things they do to help cleanse our body. Learn which foods boost immunity or improve digestive health.

Get advice from a nutritionist like myself to put you on the right path and learn what changes you can make to help you achieve your healthy body. Remember that food is not "bad" or "good," therefore we want to avoid these labels. If we follow old habits and talk about a "bad" food, we end up associating ourselves with that food. Have you ever said, "I'm not going to eat that piece of cake because I am being good today."? We are not our food choices and need to break these old habits of calling ourselves good or bad because of what we eat.

Another part of mindful eating is learning to be kind to ourselves and understanding that we don't have to be perfect. Mindful eating is about focusing on what we eat over time, and on not judging ourselves and focusing on making progress, not perfection. Our old habits will still show up from time to time, and if we are unkind to ourselves, we may feel discouraged and give up altogether. Remember you are living a healthy lifestyle; you are not on a diet. If you find yourself going back to old eating habits, ask yourself why. Determine what you need to do differently and go back to setting small motivational goals.

If you feel you are "falling off the wagon" because you forgot and started eating in your old ways, just readjust and start over. No big deal and no guilt. Building strength in the gym will take time. Reaching 10,000 steps a day will take time. Building healthy habits will take time. Be patient and gentle with yourself. I don't know why, but women are so hard on ourselves. We say things to ourselves that we would never say to another person, so be kind to yourself and learn to love your body and life. Each person's journey is unique, so do not compare yourself to anyone else because this is your journey and no one else's.

On that note, if you are eating healthy and losing weight with a male partner, he will lose weight faster than you. Often women get frustrated because they are limiting their calories, exercising, and doing everything right and will lose very slowly while their male partner loses larger amounts more quickly. It is not a reflection of how hard you are trying, but on muscle mass and hormone regulation. Men have higher muscle mass, which burns more calories, and because of their hormone percentages, they will lose weight faster.

If you have anxiety around food or suffer from an eating disorder such as binge eating, please reach out to a licensed psychologist or counsellor. You do not have to do this alone; mental health professionals are there to help. In Canada, the National Eating Disorder Information Center (NEDIC) is available to provide information, resources, referrals, and support. Go to www.nedic.ca for more information. In the United States, the National Eating Disorder Association provides similar support, and you can find them at www.nationaleatingdisorders.org

Action Items:

➢ Put your *I am healthy reminders* everywhere!
➢ Learn your reason *why.*
➢ Set two short-term goals that are specific and realistic, why you want to achieve them, and your reward.
➢ Write in your journal daily.
➢ Make a list of the foods you can eat.
➢ Pick physical activities you like and make a commitment.
➢ Practice mindful eating.
➢ Determine your unhealthy eating triggers and make a plan.

How to Change Habits and Routines

Regardless of which dietary plan you choose to follow, changing our habits so that we don't revert to our old ways is the starting point to managing type 2 diabetes. Sounds easy, right? I'm not going to lie to you, it isn't, at least not in the beginning. But it does get easier. It is going to take effort and planning on your part until it becomes a habit. In order to manage type 2 diabetes, you will need to stay on a healthy eating plan for life or risk your health issues returning.

We are all creatures of habit. The way we brush our teeth, which sock we put on first, how we tie our shoes, even the direction we drive to work are all habits. Our brain is very efficient and has developed pathways so that we don't have to think about things. We just do them. This is great if we have healthy habits, but it makes it harder to change our unhealthy habits because it takes conscious effort. But don't worry, it can be done if you put the effort in.

They say (whoever *they* are) it takes thirty days to make a new habit. Personally, I have found it takes three or more months before this way of eating becomes a lifestyle and you don't have to think about it anymore. Don't be discouraged though—by following this plan and the tips I am providing below; you can make the necessary changes to have an amazingly healthy active life.

In the beginning you will find that writing out your menu plan, tracking your food (and how it impacts your glucose levels), and having an accountability partner are helpful tools. We need reminders to keep us working toward our goal when we first begin a new lifestyle. Perhaps you wish for a friend or family member follow this plan with you. You may wish to track your success in a journal or online with your support group. Food can be tracked using an online program such as Chronometer, or My Fitness App. Most of these are free and can be used to track calories, macronutrients, set goals, and can be shared with your doctor or nutritionist. You can even input recipes, so you don't have to input the same information over and over again.

Be sure you choose to share your journey with those who will support you in a kind manner. An accountability partner who is negative, unkind, or who allows you to use old excuses for not changing habits will not help you in the long term. Be clear on how this person is going to support you, remind you of your goals, and talk to you when you are heading back into old habits. We may all think we need a Gillian Michaels to yell at us and keep us on the straight and narrow, but let's be honest, how are you going to react to that? If your support buddy makes a comment about the bag of chips you want to eat, how will you respond? Will you say, "Oh, thanks for reminding me," or will you be more like an "I will eat what I want. Stop nagging at me!" kind of person? By talking about the type of support you want and need and being very clear on the messaging, you can establish some healthy boundaries that will assist you but won't make your support buddy feel like the bad guy. You will also want to have your doctor, and nutritionist, or dietician as part of your support group.

As I explained in the introduction, changing our habits is key to creating a healthy lifestyle and managing type 2 diabetes. But it does not do you any good if I tell you to change your habits and routines but do not tell you *how* to change them. The first step is adjusting our mindset, and the second is creating new habits. We are all creatures of habit, which sometimes is a good thing and other times not so much.

Neuroscientists have discovered that every habit has three parts: the first is the "cue" that tells our brains to go into automatic mode; the second is the routine or action; and the third is the reward that makes our brain want to do the behavior again. They have discovered habits are made in the basal ganglia part of the brain, while decisions are made in the prefrontal cortex.

Once we have repeated a behavior a few times, it becomes automatic, which is helpful for allowing us to complete other tasks or thoughts at the same time. This is why we can have a conversation on the phone at the same time as folding laundry. We tend to perform these automatic tasks the same way: we put our shoes on the same foot first, we brush our teeth on the same side first, we sit the same way, and we dress the same way. Habits are built through learning and repetition and become an impulse that we no longer think about. Sometimes, these habits are handy! They allow us to multi-task or free up our brain for other things. But sometimes these habits can be bad for us. Have you ever driven to work and then realized you have no memory of actually driving there? Or made popcorn for a movie but you aren't even hungry?

The best way to break a habit is to create an entirely new environment. Believe it or not, the best time to change your diet is while on vacation, when your regular routine is not available. I know you are probably thinking, *"But Shawn, I want to relax when I am on vacation!"* I'm not telling you not to enjoy your holidays, but creating a different environment is key to breaking old habits.

Breaking bad habits can be difficult because we may not even be aware that we have them; it requires some conscious thinking about our day-to-day actions to identify the cues and rewards that create your habits. For example, if you love to eat chicken nuggets, then the cue may be the smell and the reward the taste. If you want to avoid chicken nuggets, how can you avoid the cue? Perhaps you need to avoid restaurants that serve them or not buy them for your house?

When we decide to change a habit, the first thing to do is identify the habit you wish to change and the new habit you wish to create. Decide how you will remind yourself (because you will revert to old habits) and how you will reward yourself for the new behavior (but not with food). Finally, implement the change and if you mess up, just start over. It will take several attempts before you successfully create a new habit.

Ways to create healthy habits are very dependent on the individual, but here are some suggestions that might get you started. Choose the ones that will work for you and your situation:

❖ Put post-it notes on the bathroom mirror, the car stereo, your computer, or anywhere that will remind you of your goal. Put reminders on your phone and computer.

❖ Avoid places you might be tempted. If you always drive by a fast-food restaurant and the smell tempts you, take another route.

❖ Avoid activities that might tempt you. For example, if you eat chips while watching television at night, then either don't watch television or find an alternative snack.

❖ Put yourself in situations where you are more likely to engage in your desired behavior. Hang out with people who have healthy habits.

❖ Build in incentives or rewards, but make sure the rewards are not food or drink.

❖ Tell someone you are breaking a habit and they need to remind you (in a gentle and kind manner), but don't get upset with them when they do.

❖ Destress, because stressful situations can push us back to old habits of consuming unhealthy foods and drinks.

❖ Remember that it is not about perfection, but progress. So, if you fail, just start again. Do not think of yourself as a failure if you fail, just try again.

❖ Learn the difference between what you need and what you want. I might want a piece of apple pie, but I need an apple.

❖ Drink plenty of water and herbal teas.

❖ Keep healthy snacks in the car, at work, and in your bag so that you aren't tempted when hungry.

❖ Read food labels and learn what you are eating. Knowledge is power!

❖ Make it enjoyable. For example, if you are eating new foods that you do not care for, the final step of a habit is not in place, and you are less likely to repeat the behavior. Find foods and activities that you enjoy.

❖ Focus on the long-term goal (reducing insulin levels, losing weight, and being healthy for life) rather than the short-term goals (eating unhealthy food that tastes good for a few minutes).

❖ Get enough sleep! We make terrible choices when we are tired, and we will reach for sugary foods for energy.

❖ Plan out your menu for the week based on what your family will eat, and your lifestyle. This takes a bit of effort before it becomes a habit. Write it down and put it up where you can see it as a physical reminder. Input your food into an online tracker.

❖ Make it easy. If eating healthy and exercising is difficult, you will be less likely to do either. For example, try cooking in large batches to save time or getting rid of tempting food in the house. Wash and prep your fruits and vegetables as soon as you return from the grocery store. This way they are prepped, and you won't have any excuses later.

❖ Put the healthy foods at eye level, not buried in a drawer. We have all had those mushy green things found in the back of the fridge drawer we bought with the best of intentions, but it was forgotten until it was too late. Put the healthy stuff front and center.

❖ Do bulk cooking on your day off to help carry you through the week. For example, bake enough chicken and turkey breasts for lunches for the week and then freeze them in individual containers for use later. If you have to heat the oven and pull out the meat for cooking, why not do it all at once?

❖ Make soups or stews for later use in the week. Pre-wash vegetables and put them in containers in the fridge. This makes preparing meals much faster.

❖ Keep unsalted nuts and seeds in the house, car, and at work for a quick protein snack.

❖ Do not bring junk food into the house. If you do not have quick access to it, by the time you go and buy it, the temptation may have passed.

❖ Watching television will promote eating, probably from all the food commercials we see. This is especially true for children. Advertisements for colorful cereals, cookies, snack boxes, etc. are targeted toward children. Cut back on the amount of television you watch.

❖ Only buy the food on your grocery list to avoid temptation shopping. Unless you have forgotten toilet paper, stick to your list.

❖ Eat before you go to the store. There is nothing worse than walking into the grocery store with your tummy growling as you smell the fresh baked bread or cookies. I know I have bought more stuff than I need, and not the healthiest choices, because I went shopping hungry.

❖ When you go to a restaurant, ask the waiter to skip the breadbasket. These baskets are filled with white flour high-sugar products that will spike your insulin.

❖ Order first at a restaurant so you are not tempted by someone else's poor decision.

❖ If it is a big meal, ask for a takeaway box right away and put half in the container out of sight. If the waitress won't bring the box until the end, get up and ask another staff member for one.

❖ Look at the menu online before you go in order to determine whether there are healthier options while you are not as hungry. Then don't even open the menu when you arrive. When I do this, I am not as tempted by the other items when I get there.

❖ Always have protein or healthy fat with your carbohydrates. This will slow the rise and absorption of glucose and keep insulin levels lower.

❖ Keep a journal of the foods you eat, and your blood sugar levels if you are using a glucose monitor. This will allow you to track foods that raise your blood sugar.

❖ Skip the breakfast cereal and have oatmeal with berries and 1 tbsp of ground flaxseed or scrambled eggs with vegetables, or a green smoothie made with whole fruit, leafy greens, ground flaxseed, and avocados.

❖ Be prepared. I know it sounds like the Boy Scout motto, but not being prepared means you will reach for those packaged instant foods when you are hungry and looking for something to eat. Whether you are travelling on vacation, driving home from work, stuck in the office working overtime, or sitting at home watching television, being prepared with healthy food options is key to switching to a healthy lifestyle.

Now you have some ideas on how to make healthy changes and how to keep yourself on track, implement the ones that will work for you. Obviously, you don't want to make all the changes at once or it might be too overwhelming. Pick two or three to start with and, when you are comfortable with those, add in a few more. Change can be overwhelming but with the right motivation and reminders, it is possible.

Support is very important when making changes and whether you choose a friend, join a local support group, Facebook group, or other online program, getting the support and answers you need is important. Support groups help us to feel less alone and allow us to ask questions or vent in a safe place if we need to. Please remember that chat groups provide personal opinions and anecdotal evidence, not medical advice. Always check with your doctor to ensure the information is right for you.

Saboteurs are people who encourage us to deviate from our healthy lifestyle. They might be your partner, who brings home your favorite junk food, or your friend, who wants you to skip your workout and just hang out instead. Sometimes, they are a family member who feels threatened by the changes you are making. Normally, a saboteur is not doing this out of malice, but out of fear of change or ignorance. You need to be able to identify these people and have a plan to communicate with them. Be understanding but stand your ground. Explain that you are still the same person, but want to be a healthier, happier, more energetic person that will be around for years to come. Encourage them to talk to you about their fears and feelings.

Sometimes, we need to avoid certain people who won't stop sabotaging our healthy living efforts. You might have a friend or co-worker who constantly brings in "treats" even though you have spoken to them about this. Or maybe you have a relative that always wants you to eat more because it is culturally accepted. I'm not saying cut that person out of your life completely but do set boundaries to protect your healthy lifestyle. At least until you feel strong enough to deal with them.

Action Items:

➤ Identify the cues and rewards of your habits.
➤ Choose and implement at least five of the tips.
➤ Identify your support partners and talk to them about your healthy life plan.

General Nutrition Information

The next step to managing type 2 diabetes is changing our dietary intake to lower blood glucose, improve digestive health, and create a healthier lifestyle.

All calories are not created equal. It isn't just how many calories we eat but what our body does with these that counts. For example, if we eat fibrous foods, some of the fibre goes to feed the bacteria in our digestive system (soluble fibre), and the rest of the fibre (the insoluble fibre) is used to bulk up stool (yup, I'm talking about poop) and remove toxins and waste from our body. Here, although we are *eating* calories, we aren't *absorbing* them. The calories from an apple would provide energy in the form of glucose and fibre, which will slow the absorption of the glucose and therefore rate of insulin production, as well as providing vitamins, phytonutrients, and minerals. But if we eat a cookie instead of an apple, we will have high glucose, high insulin, no fibre, no vitamins, no minerals, and poor fats. These calories will contribute to ill health.

Focusing on nutritious whole foods give us greater nutrition for fewer calories with lower glucose levels. These are foods such as leafy greens, sprouts, vegetables, berries, fruit, lean hormone-free proteins, and whole natural grains. When we eat foods that are nutritious, we provide our body the vitamins, minerals, phytonutrients, and fibre it needs to heal and re-balance, while processed food provides nothing more than empty calories and high glucose levels.

There is no "one size fits all" when it comes to dietary plans. It is a personal choice based on comfort levels, food availability, health issues, weight, doctor recommendations, and culture. There are two dietary programs I recommend for you, and I will outline the pros and cons to both of them later in the book. You may choose to try them both and see which works best for you, or you may rotate between the two. Before starting any new health program, be sure to consult your doctor.

I am going to provide you with some basic nutrition information on carbohydrates, lentils, proteins, and fats. Understanding how each of these macronutrients supports and nourishes the body will help you create the best dietary plan for your needs.

Carbohydrates

Carbohydrates are the main source of blood glucose and therefore the body's fastest, and only, energy source for the brain and red blood cells. Carbohydrates are found in grains, fruits, vegetables, dairy, berries, and melons and are divided into two types: simple and complex. Simple carbs include fructose (fruit sugar), sucrose (table sugar), and lactose (milk sugar).

Complex carbs are also made of sugars. In these, however, the molecules are strung together to form longer and more complex chains and are broken down into two types of carbohydrates: starch (grains, potatoes, beans), and fibre (leafy greens and vegetables). Starch and sugar are both broken down into glucose in the body and fibre passes through the body (insoluble fibre) or feeds our digestive system (soluble fibre). These are the foods that provide us energy when glucose enters our blood stream.

Without carbohydrates, we would not be able to obtain the essential vitamins, minerals, and phytonutrients we need for optimal health. Our brain, red blood cells, kidneys, and central nervous system prefers carbohydrates to any other type of fuel.

Dietary fibre, sometimes called roughage, is a very important form of carbohydrate that comes from the part of the plant that does not break down when in contact with our digestive enzymes. As a result, only a small amount is metabolized in our intestines, with most of it moving through our intestinal tract and delivering important health benefits. Fibre retains water, which results in softer, bulkier stool (poop), helping prevent constipation and/or hemorrhoids. Scientists believe fibre helps reduce the risk of colon cancer because it moves stool faster through intestine and keeps the digestive tract clean.

Another health benefit is that fibre binds with substances that would result in the production of cholesterol and helps remove them from the body, which helps lower cholesterol levels and reduce the risk of heart disease. All hormones are made from cholesterol and recent studies suggest that women with PCOS, insulin resistance, and thyroiditis benefit from reducing cholesterol through a high-fibre diet.

Clinical and experimental studies all show that people with type 2 diabetes tend to be low in dietary fibre intake. Different types of fibre have different benefits in the body, with soluble fibre having the greatest benefit for blood sugar control. These fibres slow down the digestion and absorption of glucose, therefore slowing the rise of blood sugar levels. Soluble fibres also increase the sensitivity of tissues to insulin, therefore improving the absorption of glucose by the muscles, liver, and other tissues. Great examples of soluble fibre include apples, oat bran, nuts, seeds, pears, and most vegetables.

High fibre foods help protect the liver and feed the healthy bacteria in our digestive system, allowing for better absorption of nutrients, helping fight many types of cancer, and ensuring the proper elimination of waste. A healthy liver will remove excess hormones, insulin, and toxins from our system, however excess sugar, alcohol, processed foods, and high levels of omega-6 fatty acids will negatively impact our liver, slowing the removal of excess insulin, toxins, and waste. Fibre is our friend! Please note, I am talking about natural fibre from fruits, berries, nuts, seeds, and vegetables, not the fibre supplement powder that has become so popular in society today. Supplement powders do not work the same way in our body, lack nutrition, and do not feed the good bacteria in our digestive system. Skip the powder and eat real food! By adding fiber to every meal, we can reduce the glycemic load (the measure of how quickly a food raises glucose levels) and improve our overall health. Fiber is the most important food to add to your diet for better health.

Glucose is either used immediately for energy, or a small portion is stored in the liver for future use (which is why you still have energy hours after eating). However, if we consume more calories than our body requires, we will store this extra glucose as adipose tissue (fat cells), which will be stored in our liver (contributing to non-alcoholic fatty liver disease), and around our organs (visceral fat) as well as under the skin (subcutaneous fat).

Scientists believe this is a genetic feature that allows us to survive in times of famine, or when we do not have regular access to food. This is especially important for women due to the demanding physical needs of pregnancy and nursing. While a hundred years ago this was a great genetic trait to have, in modern times with our easy access to food, it can be frustrating. This is why it is important to stay within the caloric needs of your body.

The glycemic index is a measure of how quickly a food causes our blood sugar levels to rise after eating, the higher the number, the greater the blood sugar response. This means a low GI food will cause a small rise, while a high GI food will cause a rise. A GI of 70 or more is high, a GI of 56 to 69 is medium, and a GI of 55 or less is considered low. There are a number of factors that affect the glycemic index of a food, such as the type of sugar it contains, the structure of the starch, and how refined the carbohydrate is; even the ripeness can change the glycemic index rating. Complex carbohydrates tend to, but don't always, have a lower number; some simple carbohydrates have a higher number.

The glycemic load is a classification of foods with carbohydrates that measures the impact on the body and blood sugar. It's used to help you understand how high your blood sugar could go when you actually eat the food. This measurement also lets you know how much glucose per serving a particular food is providing, making it a slightly better tool for people with insulin dependent diabetes.

Fruit juice is a great example of the glycemic load. Whole fruit contains fibre which slows down the absorption of the glucose, keeping our insulin levels lower. While fruit juice is pure sugar, it does not contain the fibre or phytonutrients that provide health benefits and creates a spike in glucose, and therefore insulin. Avoid fruit juice, fruit punch, or fruit-flavored drinks and eat whole fruit instead.

Whether you choose to use the glycemic index or glycemic load, reducing the glycemic (sugar) levels of the foods you eat and adding in more fibre will help to lower blood sugar levels. I have provided a list at the end of the book to help you get started. This list is not exhaustive, so refer to the internet if you are unsure. There are many glycemic index or glycemic load cheat sheets available to you and after a while you will learn which foods to eat and which to avoid. Remember, by adding in fiber from vegetables or leafy greens to every meal, you can reduce the glycemic load of a meal.

Tracking carbohydrates is important when you have insulin resistance or type 2 diabetes. Some carbs can cause your blood glucose levels to spike, while others have little or no effect. There are several online apps you can use to track your food consumption, such as Chronometer (my favourite), My Fitness Pal, One Touch, and Carb Manager. Tracking your food intake and blood glucose levels will allow you to understand which foods have the most impact.

Remember that if we do not use the glucose we eat for immediate energy, our body stores the excess as fat cells. You need to understand that fat loves to store hormones and therefore the more fat we have, the more imbalanced our hormones become. Adipose tissue (fat) collects leptin (our appetite-control hormone) rather than letting it flow through the blood stream to the brain to tell us we are full. This is why we keep eating and thinking we are hungry despite having had sufficient food.

Adipose tissue also produces estrogen, which can create estrogen dominance. Symptoms of estrogen dominance include heavy painful periods, decreased sex drive, bloating, mood swings, fatigue, breast tenderness, fibroids, and hormonal weight gain. Keeping our glucose levels low will allow us to keep our insulin levels low and keeping our insulin levels low will reduce our adipose tissue, which will in turn help to balance our hormones. Study after study has shown that weight loss has been helpful in managing type 2 diabetes.

Recent studies have shown that processed foods may be the cause of many health-related illnesses and disease. As our rates of processed food consumption have risen, so have the rates of obesity, diabetes, and heart disease. Coincidence? I don't think so. I know it might be a bit challenging to remove these foods as they are widely available, cheap, and have become a big part of our daily diet. Start by removing the obvious ones (the ones we call junk food), and then slowly remove the others one at a time. You will need to find alternatives in your diet for these foods. For example, have salad or soup instead of a sandwich. Have an apple with peanut butter for a snack instead of a bag of potato chips. Skip the toast for breakfast and have scrambled eggs with vegetables, oatmeal with berries, or a green smoothie.

White bread products should be avoided at all costs! They are highly processed (the flour is bleached to give it that smooth, light appearance), have little nutritional value, contain high amounts of sugar, and lead to high spikes in blood sugar, which will cause it to crash, making us reach for more food. White bread products can cause bloating, acid reflux, and constipation because it does not break down properly in our body. Foods that are high in sugar also contain addictive qualities that have us reaching for more, and studies have shown that highly-refined carbohydrates are linked to poor digestive and mental health, and anxiety.

Whole grains, such as ancient grains (millet, quinoa, spelt, barley, bulgur, amaranth, rye, or brown rice), can be healthy. While grains contain fibre, which slows the absorption of glucose and is good for the digestive system,

I recommend avoiding wheat as it has been shown to cause sensitivities in many people, as well as raising cholesterol, disrupting blood sugar levels, can cause leaky gut, bloating and gas, and is always mixed with sugar in food products. Modern wheat comes from GMO seeds created to resist insects and are exposed to high numbers of pesticides and fertilizers. The wheat is then ground, separated from the bran, and then refortified to try and replace the vitamins and minerals that were removed during the processing. Wheat contains a protein called wheat germ agglutinin, which keeps us from absorbing nutrients over time. As Dr. Mark Hyman notes, "because wheat has been genetically modified, it now contains a super-starch called Amylopectin A that causes wheat (whole grain or not) to spike your blood sugar like never before."

The difficulty with removing bread products is they are everywhere and very convenient. Go into any gas station and you will find row upon row of brightly packaged cookies, crackers, doughnuts, and muffins. Fast food restaurants provide sandwiches, buns, burgers, tacos, and pizza. Removing bread products can be difficult for many people as they have become a staple in our diet. Two pieces of toast for breakfast, a sandwich for lunch, a roll with dinner and we have just consumed five servings of bread, while the recommended serving is one. Yes, you read that correctly. One serving. One slice of bread, 1/2 bagel, or one small dinner roll is the recommended amount. It is no wonder that as a society we are getting sicker and fatter. Just removing the excess bread products will have a positive impact on our weight and our blood sugar levels.

Breakfast cereals are a quick easy food for breakfast, especially for kids who can pour their own in the morning. I get it! But are we doing ourselves or our children any favors? The problem with breakfast cereals is the high sugar content. Cereals can have over 50% sugar content! Sugar is usually listed as the second or third ingredient and many cereals contain multiple types of sugar. Highly refined flours have little to no nutritional value, but these products are often marketed to children with brightly colored boxes, marshmallows, cartoon characters, or action figures. The high sugar content causes a massive increase in glucose/insulin, followed by a crash. Sugar is addictive and after eating just a small amount, we want more. And, let's be honest, no one eats the 3/4 cup serving size of cereal. We grab a bowl and fill it up, which may equal three or four servings rather than one. Try serving plain cheerios, which are gluten-free and low in sugar, eggs with vegetables, or oatmeal with berries for breakfast.

Unprocessed carbohydrates are foods containing only one ingredient. They may be a grain, such as quinoa or barley, or they can be a fruit, berry, melon, or vegetable. If you look at the list of ingredients, only one food is listed. These foods are consumed in their most natural state. As I mentioned earlier, they provide soluble and insoluble fibre to reduce cholesterol and improve digestion. Grains and complex carbohydrates (such as sweet potatoes) also provide a heaviness to the meal that helps keep us feeling full. My grandma used to serve us oatmeal in the morning because it would "stick to your ribs." And while it doesn't *actually* stick to your ribs, it does help us feel fuller longer. When you change your diet to reduce large intakes of bread products and increase intake of vegetables and unprocessed grain such as rice or quinoa, or root vegetables such as sweet potato, it will help with feeling fuller longer, so you don't feel hungry and tempted to cheat.

Unprocessed grains such as oatmeal, wheat, and barley may contain gluten—which is a common sensitivity for many people. If these foods cause excessive gas or bloating, reduce, or eliminate them. You may find that one grain causes bloating while another does not. Brown and wild rice and quinoa do not contain gluten, so these may be a better option for you.

Sprouts are little powerhouses of nutrition. They are seeds that have sprouted but are not yet plants. There are many different types of sprouts, including: alfalfa, quinoa, pea, broccoli, green pea, and more. They contain high levels of folate, magnesium, phosphorus, niacin, riboflavin, zinc, iron, calcium, and Vitamin K. Alfalfa, quinoa, and soybean sprouts are also a great source of protein for vegetarians and vegans. Sprouts contain high levels of enzymes and are therefore good for our digestion. Enzymes are a key part of the digestive system as they help break down food and may help increase the absorption of nutrients from the digestive tract. In addition, sprouts contain dietary fibre which helps to bulk up the stool, allowing it to pass more easily through the digestive tract. Additionally, they may help boost our metabolism because of the high level of enzymes and nutrients.

A word of caution, there have been cases of food poisoning linked to sprouts so be sure to wash them thoroughly and/or cook before eating, especially for those at high risk such as pregnant women, children, the elderly, or those with a weakened immunity. I like to wash mine, spin them dry in a salad spinner, and then store in a container that allows air flow to keep them from going mushy.

Leafy greens such as romaine lettuce, green and red leafy lettuce, arugula, spinach, beet tops, collard greens, and kale are low in calories and high in folates, fiber, vitamin A, C, and K, as well as magnesium, iron, and potassium. They contain many antioxidants and have anti-inflammatory properties. Leafy greens have been shown to help reduce blood pressure, aid in weight loss, reduce cholesterol, and help prevent heart disease. Please note that if you are taking any type of blood thinner, you need to speak with your doctor if you are eating a large number of foods with vitamin K, as it helps to clot the blood. I understand that you may not want to eat non-stop salads, especially in the winter months, so I have included the recipe for a Green Smoothie which is a fabulous way to get your fruits and fibre. If you have never tried a green smoothie, don't worry, you only taste the fruit!

Vegetables grown above the ground tend to have lower glucose levels than those we call "root vegetables." Vegetables provide fibre, vitamins, minerals, phytonutrients, and have been shown to be the most effective tool in fighting high insulin levels. There are hundreds of different types of vegetables grown around the world all providing us with the nutrition we need to be healthy. Try different vegetables or recipes to expand your tastes and avoid food boredom.

I have referred to phytonutrients a few times in this book and would be remiss if I didn't explain what they are. Phytonutrients are thousands of organic compounds within a plant food that provide powerful antioxidants that protect our cells. Many phytonutrients have been shown to reduce the risk of cancer, heart disease, stroke, Alzheimer's, and Parkinson's disease. They boost our immune system, lower inflammation in our body and studies have shown them to be very helpful to diabetics. Phytonutrients are found in the colour, taste, aroma, and texture of a plant food. Increasing our intake of phytonutrients may end up being the most important change we can make in our diet.

Legumes, beans, lentils

Legumes, beans, peas, and lentils are complex carbohydrates that contain protein, fibre, and minerals and tend to have little effect on blood glucose levels. Many are naturally gluten-free and low in calories. A study published in the journal JAMA found that people who included legumes, beans, and lentils in their diet had better glycemic control and a lower risk of heart disease. They slow digestion and therefore the absorption of glucose, which keeps insulin from spiking. They are also low on the glycemic index, filling, high in fibre (good for bowels), fairly inexpensive, and can be bought in bulk. Additionally, they are also a great source of protein, potassium, folate, iron, magnesium, and calcium. They contain resistant starch (food for the good bacteria in our digestive system) and therefore support a healthy digestive system.

Legumes, beans, peas, and lentils are considered an incomplete protein (meaning they lack one or more amino acids) so it is important to add a complementary protein (a food that has the lacking amino acid) to make a complete protein. It sounds complicated, but it really isn't.

e.g.

- Combine beans with either brown rice, nuts, seeds, wheat, or corn.
- Combine brown rice with beans, nuts, or seeds.
- Combine peas with nuts, seeds, or wild rice to get a complete protein.

To incorporate these into your diet, some examples of menu items are peanut butter on whole wheat toast, beans and rice, hummus and pita bread, refried beans and corn tortillas, or salad with chickpeas and seeds.

If you are put off from including beans in your diet because of the preparation time, there's no need to worry. The old method of soaking beans overnight then slow cooking them for hours to soften them up is no longer required. An Insta Pot can cook beans from dry to ready in about seventy-five minutes. You may want to cook a large batch then freeze the cooked beans to use later, or make up large batches of soups, chilis, or casseroles and freeze those instead.

Avoid canned beans, as many cans contain BPA (an endocrine disruptor that may imbalance hormones) and have added salt and sugar that you want to avoid. Dry beans are much cheaper than canned, take up less room in the pantry and are more nutritious. A bag of dried kidney beans can be purchased for only a couple of dollars (less at a discount store or bought in bulk), while a single can of kidney beans can be $1.48, which adds up very quickly if you want to include these nutritious foods in your diet.

Overall, it is more important to change the type of carbohydrates we eat than focusing on the amount we eat. By removing processed carbohydrates that include sugar, high fructose corn syrup, white flour and loads of preservatives and artificial flavourings and adding in more natural carbohydrates in the form of fresh vegetables, leafy greens, beans, nuts, seeds, and natural grains; we can drastically improve our health.

Protein

Protein is essential for growth, healing, manufacturing hormones, muscles, skin, hair, and helps make antibodies that fight infection and illness. When we consume protein, our body breaks the food down into amino acids. Some amino acids are essential (meaning we have to eat them), while others are nonessential (meaning our body can create them by joining other amino acids together). Dietary proteins are divided into two groups: complete proteins (found in fish, poultry, cheese, eggs, soybeans, and dairy), and incomplete proteins (found in grains, legumes, and leafy green vegetables).

Lean protein includes beans, nuts, soy, fish, seafood, poultry, and eggs. When combined with a carbohydrate, protein helps to slow absorption of glucose, which keeps insulin lower and provides satiety. This doesn't mean you should go crazy for meat products, as high protein levels have an insulinotropic effect as they promote insulin secretion and may promote heart disease, as they are higher in saturated fats.

There is a myth that we can never have too much protein. This myth has supported the marketing efforts of protein powders, pills, and diets around the world. But something you need to understand is that "protein" isn't stored in the body. All protein is broken down in the body into amino acids and absorbed in the small intestine. These amino acids are then sent through the blood stream to various parts of the body for cell repair, hormone synthesis, and building muscle. If we eat more than our body needs, it will be broken down into glycogen, then into glucose, and ultimately be stored as fat.

Eating extra protein will not help build bigger muscles faster or make us stronger. People with a higher metabolism (such as athletes or body builders) have a higher need for protein than the average person. These people may take protein powders to "build up" muscle, as the amount of protein they need to consume would have their triglycerides and cholesterol through the roof. But unless you are an athlete or a body builder, you can stick to three servings of protein a day in the correct portion sizes.

The protein you should consume will consist of wild-caught fish to increase your omega-3 fatty acids, organic hormone free eggs, hormone-free organic chicken breast or turkey, lean hormone-free grass-fed beef, and hormone-free organic pork. Seeing a trend here? In order to balance our hormones naturally, it is important to reduce or remove all the added hormones that are often found in meat products.

Studies are "inconclusive" about whether the hormones given to animals influence our health, but I believe constantly bombarding our body with hormones and toxins will have a negative lasting effect. Studies have shown that women with insulin resistance may be more sensitive to these hormones, and so removing them keeps the body from having to deal with any possible additional stress. Additionally, animals that are fed corn as their main food source have much higher rates of omega-6 fatty acids, creating an imbalance with our omega-3 fatty acids and leading to inflammation and disease in the body. By eating hormone free, grass fed, organic meat, we avoid excess hormones and maintain a healthier balance of our omega fats. I will explain more about healthy fats later in the book.

Studies have shown that tofu and other vegetarian protein options, such as lentils or beans, help to reduce saturated fats, androgens (which cause some symptoms of polycystic ovary syndrome), lower cholesterol, reduce risks of heart disease and stroke, and provide more fibre to aid in elimination. Eating vegetarian options may not only lower your grocery bill but help balance hormones as well.

In a study from the University of Alabama, it showed that women who were omnivores (ate meat, poultry, fish, vegetables, and fruit) had a higher BMI, higher rates of type 2 diabetes and higher risk of heart disease compared to women who were vegetarian, semi-vegetarian (they ate vegetarian three times a week), or vegan. Women in the study who ate semi-vegetarian, vegetarian, or vegan lost a higher percentage of weight than the omnivores. Over a six-month period, the vegan group lost the most weight, followed by the vegetarians and semi-vegetarians, and finally, the omnivores.

The study clearly indicated eating a plant-based diet allowed for greater weight loss and the prevention and treatment of obesity-related diseases. Full disclosure, the results could have been because they removed processed food and instead ate real food with fibre and nutrients, rather than the removal of meat. But either way, vegetable foods are clearly a healthier option. Now, I am not telling you that you must become vegan or vegetarian but consider adding more vegetables to your diet to improve your health.

Canadian researchers have discovered soybeans, chickpeas, peas, and lentils contain natural components that seem to work at the cellular level to reduce insulin resistance and block body fat storage. They did an experiment asking women to have two cups of unsweetened plain soymilk daily, or seven ounces of tofu for twelve weeks. At the end of the experiment, the number of androgens (male hormones that promote belly fat) in their body had reduced along with insulin resistance. Some women find this helpful while others do not. I recommend you try soy products first and see how you react.

Like many other products, soy was once considered a diet food and was added to every processed product so that it could be promoted as "healthy." Not all soy is the same. Because of its rise in popularity during the fad-diet phase, many companies began using cheap, nonorganic soy that did not contain the same health benefits. Look for organic unsweetened soy products in the most unprocessed form.

Remove all processed meats including deli meats (salami, bacon, ham, pepperoni, jerky, packaged lunch meats), preformed meats (fish sticks, spam, and chicken nuggets), and high fat meats. Processed meats contain high amounts of salt, which can cause bloating and water retention as well as containing added preservative nitrates.

Studies show that nitrates may increase risk of colon cancer, heart disease, and create an added load on the liver. Remember the liver is the cleaning powerhouse of the body and we want to eat as cleanly as possible to reduce its load, allowing more toxins and extra hormones to be removed from the body. Highly-processed foods are also highly inflammatory in the body, so the removal of processed meats will reduce inflammation. High inflammation equals higher chance of disease.

Studies have shown that nuts provide beneficial monounsaturated and polyunsaturated fats that improve insulin sensitivity, are rich in fibre and magnesium, and have a low glycemic index. One Brazil nut contains the required daily amount of selenium. Pumpkin seeds contain zinc which helps create a strong immune system, as well as vitamins and minerals such as manganese which aid in wound healing. Almonds are high in unsaturated fatty acids and minerals that help to protect our heart. Walnuts have a high amount of omega-3 fatty acids and are great for our brain health. These are just a few examples, but as you can see, nuts and seeds are good for our health and make a great snack option but can be highly caloric, so eat only a 1/4 cup daily.

We all know the slogan "milk, it does a body good," and if you are like me, you grew up drinking milk and eating dairy products because you were told it would give you calcium for strong bones. The problem is that dairy contains casein and lactose, and over fifty percent of adults cannot digest these proteins properly, which can cause stomach upset, gas, bloating, diarrhea, and inflammation.

Milk is the most common food allergy and the most underreported. There have been studies indicating that milk has a negative correlation with insulin sensitivity and insulin resistance. Basically, the higher the intake of dairy, the higher the rate of insulin resistance. Whether or not you choose to believe the reports on the overuse of antibiotics and hormones given to dairy cows, or the treatment of animals in some farms, the fact dairy causes so many digestive issues should have you considering other options.

If you grew up on milk products, like I did, it may take some adjustment to find alternatives. I still prefer to use a small amount of unsalted butter in my diet over margarine, as butter contains butyric acid and feeds the cells in the large intestine. Margarine is a hydrogenated product and studies have shown it does not provide any health benefits. Soy milk, almond milk, and oat milk are a few options if you want to keep milk in your diet. Rice milk is high in the glycemic index and therefore not recommended. Processed cheese and cheese spreads are often higher in fat and sodium, but I have found some delicious organic goat cheese that I use on special occasions, because goat milk contains less lactose than cows' milk, is easier to digest, has fewer calories, is rich in vitamins and minerals, and goats tend to be treated more humanely. But do check your labels, some imported cheese does not meet the same standards.

Ice cream has the highest rates of fat congestion and highest sugar content among dairy products. It may be both the greatest joy and the greatest threat to our health because it is cheap, widely available, and is considered a special treat. It is served at children's birthday parties, and parents take great delight in giving their toddlers their first taste of ice cream. Please reserve ice cream for those rare occasions and do not give it to toddlers. Ice cream has a lot of preservatives, sweeteners, artificial colors, and flavours which can cause abdominal discomfort and diarrhea. Children under twenty-four months should avoid foods high in sugars as they are linked to obesity and cavities and may in fact start a lifelong addiction to sweets.

Fats

Eating healthy fat does not make you fat. Let's just get that out of the way. Up to the age of two we have a higher requirement for fat in our diet as our bodies need fat for normal brain development, but as an adult we require at least twenty-five to thirty percent of our diet to consist of healthy fats. As adults, we need it to absorb fat-soluble vitamins, and for healthy hair, skin, joints, and eyes. Dietary fat helps our cells communicate, our nerves send messages to the brain, our glands make hormones, and our body transport vitamins where they are needed.

I can always tell when a person has been following a low-fat diet as healthy-fat deficiency symptoms include dry skin, mood swings, depression, hormone imbalance, poor vitamin absorption, increased sensitivity to light, easy bruising, loose teeth, muscle pain, heart palpitations, fatigue, aching joints, and brain fog. Once healthy fats are reintroduced in proper portions, these symptoms go away. Notice I am talking about healthy fats, not manmade trans-fat, or hydrogenated fats.

While we do need to keep an eye on our total quantity of fats to stay within our caloric needs, the *quality* of the fats we consume is more important. Fatty acids are basically like links in a chain made up of carbon atoms. There are short-chain fatty acids (two to five links), medium-chain fatty acids (six to twelve) and long-chain fatty acids (fourteen to eighteen), and our body needs all three types to remain healthy.

We categorize fats by their degree of saturation of hydrogen molecules. There are three main categories: saturated, polyunsaturated, and monounsaturated, based on the number of hydrogen atoms in the chemical structure of a given molecule of fatty acid. To remain healthy, we need both saturated and unsaturated fatty acids. While we categorize a food or oil as saturated, polyunsaturated, or monounsaturated, in reality most foods are a combination of these fatty acids, and we categorize based on the predominant one.

Saturated fats are normally solid at room temperature and are found in animal products such as meat, cheese, and butter. Some cuts of meat are higher in saturated fats, such as pork, ham, beef, veal, and lamb. You can tell from the marbling how much saturated fat is in the product. Just as a side note, animals raised on corn or other fatty acids high in omega-6 will have heavy marbling in the center and edges of the cut of meat. Wild meat or organic grass-fed meat will have smaller lines and may have slightly darker meat. Coconut and palm kernel oil are also high in saturated fat. We do need some saturated fat in our diet as our liver uses this to manufacture cholesterol (which we use to create hormones), however excess intake will raise our LDL (bad cholesterol), which promotes heart disease.

Polyunsaturated fatty acids are found in corn, soybeans, safflower, sunflower oils, some nuts and seeds, and some fish oils. Polyunsaturated fats are high in calories and may lower levels of HDL (good cholesterol). Therefore, experts tell us no more than ten percent of the total calories consumed should come from this group. Fish (salmon, mackerel, tuna, herring, and sardines) and seeds and nuts (flaxseeds, chia seeds, and walnuts) are also omega-3 fatty acids which science has shown do not affect our cholesterol levels and may reduce the risk of heart disease. We need some polyunsaturated fatty acids in our diet, so focus on eating fish, nuts, and seeds as part of a healthy diet.

Monounsaturated fatty acids are found mostly in nut oils such as olive, peanut, and canola oil. Scientists believe these oils reduce our LDL (bad cholesterol) without impacting our HDL (good cholesterol).

Hydrogenated fats were created to increase the shelf-life of processed foods. This process involves placing a canister of hydrogen gas below a vat of oil and allowing the gas to bubble up into the oil, which makes the oil absorb more hydrogen and unsaturated fatty acids can be changed into saturated ones called "trans fats." This process produces a semi-solid fat that is less likely to go rancid. This all sounds great, but sadly hydrogenation lowers the quality of the oil, and trans fats increase LDL cholesterol as well as the risk of atherosclerosis (hardening of the arteries). Including hydrogenated fats is what keeps bread from growing moldy after a few days, or that box of cookies on the store shelf for months. Great for the profit of the manufacturer but not for your health.

Sterols are a category of fat that includes cholesterol, phytosterols (plant sterols), and some of the steroid hormones. Cholesterol is the precursor of bile acids and sex hormones. It is made in the body, primarily in the liver, although all the bodily tissues (except the brain) can make it. Cholesterol is present in most of our cells, especially in the liver, brain, nervous tissue, and the blood. It is responsible for some of the functions that support the health of the brain, nervous system, liver, blood, and skin.

Our liver makes all the cholesterol we need to make hormones, Vitamin D and perform various other functions. The remainder in our body comes from foods such as egg yolk, meat, animal fat, and milk products but is not present in any plant foods. The liver is also responsible for removing unwanted cholesterol by converting it to bile and transferring it out of the body. We can reduce our LDL and raise our HDL levels by increasing our dietary fiber and plant phytonutrient intake, and exercise, which will reduce inflammation and oxidation in our body.

The correct ratio of omega-3 and omega-6 fatty acids helps determine the flexibility of our cell membranes (on which nearly all chemical communication throughout the body depends). Study after study has shown imbalances between omega-3 and omega-6 is linked to risk of noninsulin dependent diabetes, obesity, chronic inflammation, and heart disease.

Over the last fifty years we have been eating fewer healthy omega-3 fatty acids and a greater amount of saturated and polyunsaturated fats from corn and cottonseed oil found mostly in processed foods. We need a balance of approximately 1:1 of omega-3 fatty acids and omega-6 fatty acids, but our current North American diet containing high amounts of processed and deep-fried foods are extremely high in omega-6 but too low in omega-3 (some studies show as high as a 26:1 ratio).

Too many omega-6 fats can raise blood pressure, impact our brain health, and affect our heart. Omega-6 saturated fats increase the secretion of insulin and change the way our body uses it, which may lead to insulin resistance and atherosclerosis. In a 2016 study, Dr. Dariush Mozaffarian determined eating more unsaturated instead of saturated fats lowers both blood sugar and insulin levels. By replacing processed carbohydrates and saturated fatty foods, such as processed or fatty cuts of meat, with cold-water fish, nuts, or seeds, we can improve our metabolic health.

Balance your level of these fats by eliminating deep-fried and processed foods, by adding in wild cold-water fish two to three times per week, and through adding two tbsp of ground flaxseed to your daily diet to increase intake of healthy omega-3. Ground flaxseeds can be added to oatmeal, green smoothies, or sprinkled on salads. Eat wild fish rather than farmed fish because wild fish feed on algae that is naturally high in omega-3 fats, while farmed fish are fed corn, which is high in omega-6 fats.

We can also obtain our healthy omega-3 fats from eggs obtained from pasture-raised chickens, but not from chickens raised on corn. You can tell the difference by the color of the yolk. Grass-fed chickens that are outside eating what nature intended provide an egg with a deep yellow, almost orange-colored yolk—chickens fed corn provide an egg with a pale-yellow yolk.

When I was a young girl, my family raised chickens. The first time I bought eggs from a store when was I went away to university. I cracked the first one in the bowl and saw the pale-yellow color and thought there was something wrong with the egg, so I threw it out and cracked another one. After several eggs, I finally phoned my mother, who advised me of the difference between them.

Eliminate fried or deep-fried foods from your diet. These foods are cooked in poor quality cheap oils (usually corn oil) that raise our omega-6 fat levels, increase our cholesterol, cause heart disease, and contain excess calories we do not need. A change in the way we cook can have a big impact on our health while still allowing us to eat our favorite foods. Have baked chicken instead of fried chicken, baked potato instead of deep-fried fries, eat grass-fed meat instead of animals that were fed a diet of corn, and eat fish twice a week. You can still have stir-fried foods using a small amount of extra virgin olive oil.

A question I am often asked is about margarine versus butter. While margarine is convenient because it stays soft in the refrigerator, it is highly processed, and often contains trans fats and high amounts of salt. I have noticed that if you leave a tub on the counter, no bugs will touch it. This should tell us something! I recommend you consume unsalted butter in small amounts. Butter contains vitamins A, E, and D, as well as calcium and conjugated linoleic acid, which studies show may have anti-cancer effects and help decrease weight. Be aware that butter is highly caloric, so use it sparingly.

You may be wondering what type of oil you should be consuming or cooking with. Coconut oil contains six times more saturated fat than olive oil, and while we do need a small amount of saturated fat in our diet, I recommend avoiding high amounts of it for now. Also avoid any trans fats, hydrogenated fats, canola oil, soybean oil, or cottonseed oil. Canola oil is more pro-inflammatory while olive oil is anti-inflammatory partly due to the way they are processed because olive oil is cold-pressed while canola oil is processed using high heat and chemicals. Canola oil is also partially hydrogenated for shelf stability and can also become a trans-fat upon heating. For these reasons I recommend you use extra virgin olive oil over other oils. Please note that olive oil can also become partially hydrogenated if heated past its smoke point, so keep the temperature lower than this.

Drinks

It is important to consider what we drink as well as what we eat. If you have cream and sugar in your coffee or tea, you can easily be adding fifty calories per cup. Now, this may not sound like much, but if you drink three cups per day, that is 4,200 extra calories in one month. A McDonald's hot chocolate with whipped cream is three-hundred-and-forty calories. If you had one every week for a year, that would be 16,320 calories, or almost six extra pounds just from hot chocolate! Most blended frozen drinks at Starbucks are over three-hundred-and-forty calories and fifty-four grams of sugar cach (that's thirteen teaspoons of sugar in one drink).

Our drink choices add up very quickly. These sugary drinks can be very addictive and are part of our culture. We meet friends for coffee or grab a cup to-go, we have coffee breaks at work and many cultures also serve coffee as an after-dinner drink. In the United States over sixty-six billion cups of coffee (including espresso, latte, cappuccino, and iced coffee) are sold each year.

I love when restaurants provide the total number of calories in their drinks and the total grams of sugar, which allows us to make healthier and more informed choices, but most people don't understand "grams of sugar." A gram of sugar is hard to visualize and sounds like a tiny amount, which can be deceiving. One teaspoon equals four grams, so divide the total number of grams by four to get a better idea of how many teaspoons of sugar you are consuming. The American Heart Association recommends that men consume no more than thirty-six grams of sugar per day, and women should consume no more than twenty-five grams—for anyone with type 2 diabetes, this number is cut in half.

We need to be drinking at least six cups of water per day. If plain water is boring, or you want more variety, add a slice of lemon to your water. Hot water with a slice of lemon is a great way to start your day and can get your bowels moving. Lemon water helps to remove uric acid from joints, stimulates the liver to remove toxins, and is thought to improve digestion. If you do choose to drink lemon water, over time the acid can soften your tooth enamel, so protect your teeth by rinsing with plain water after and wait a while after your drink before you brush your teeth.

Other drinks you should consume are herbal teas such as spearmint, matcha green, or chamomile. Herbal teas support a healthy digestive and immune system, and many are loaded with antioxidants. Some are calming, others provide a great pick-me-up in the afternoon, so try several different types to see which ones you prefer. Be cautious of drinking herbal teas if you are pregnant, as some are used to induce labor and may promote a miscarriage.

Drinking enough fluids is critical for our body. We need fluids to absorb nutrients, flush out toxins, prevent constipation, balance blood pressure, and prevent cognitive problems. Even mild dehydration of 2% can create short-term memory loss, as water helps our cells communicate with each other. More extreme dehydration, or dehydration over longer periods, can create more pronounced cognitive decline as brain cells will shrink in size. This is a condition often seen in the elderly, as they are less active and therefore drink less water.

Drinking water can help to suppress our appetite, boost our metabolism, may lead to increased lipolysis (fat burning), as well as preventing constipation, and helping to flush toxins from our body. If we are working or playing in warmer temperatures, we may require more water than normal. If you are suffering from a cold or virus, drinking extra water helps to thin the mucous and get healthier faster.

Signs of dehydration can include headaches, dark urine, feeling sluggish or fatigued, extreme thirst, dry mouth, bad breath, and sugar cravings. Often, feeling thirsty is the last sign we recognize. Our urine should be the color of pale lemonade, so if the color of yours is darker, you know you need to drink more water.

It is possible to have too much of a good thing. Excessive water can also cause an imbalance in our electrolytes. If your urine is colorless, you may be drinking too much. Balance is the key! Just as a note, if you are taking supplemental B12 (riboflavin), your urine may be bright neon yellow. Nothing to panic about, B12 is a water-soluble vitamin, so your body is flushing out the excess amount. However, if you are trying to check your urine to ensure you are not dehydrated, the color will give you no indication.

As I explained earlier, drinking fruit juice or punch is not a good idea. Fruit juice lacks the fiber to slow the digestion and absorption of glucose, which causes our insulin levels to rise rapidly. Fruit punch is just sugary-flavored water with no nutritional value. If you are craving the taste of orange juice—have an orange. It will satisfy the craving and is a healthier choice than a big glass of sugary water.

Skip the soda/pop whether it is full-sugar or diet. Diet soda is worse than regular soda. Artificial sweeteners trick our body into believing we have consumed glucose, so our pancreas releases insulin. However, we now have excess insulin swimming around in our veins with no glucose. This can cause dizzy spells, sweating, anxiety, confusion, trembling hands, and if our blood sugar levels go too low, hypoglycemia. Artificial sweeteners provide no nutrition, are highly chemically-processed, and some have even been recalled because they are known carcinogens (known to cause cancer). Artificial sweeteners can be just as addictive as sugar, and have been shown to cause weight gain, bladder cancer, brain cancer, and depression.

One way to ensure you drink enough water in a day is to fill a jug with eight cups of water and try to drink it all before you go to bed at night. Or fill eight bottles to consume throughout the day. I have one client who marks their water consumption down on a piece of paper, while another uses an app on their phone. Whatever works best for you.

I recommend you keep a spare bottle of water in the car in case you are out and feeling thirsty. Keep a glass or cup at work so you have no excuse not to drink while you are there. Take a bottle with you to the gym or while on your walk. Be that person who always has a cool-looking bottle with them wherever they go. Modern plastics are BPA free, and you should look for this information before you purchase any water bottle. Many of us want to reuse our plastic water bottles from the store, which is fine for a few times, but studies indicate that the plastic will start to break down over time as it is exposed to hot water and the sun. Metal water bottles became popular for a time to reduce the amount of plastic used. I have always found that my water tastes metallic, but others use them every day with no complaints. Find what works for you.

Action Items:

- ❖ Make a list of low glycemic foods you like to eat.
- ❖ Create a weekly menu plan using the above foods and put it on the fridge.
- ❖ Create your grocery list.
- ❖ Decide how you will remind yourself to stick to your eating plan and implement it.
- ❖ Purchase a BPA-free water bottle.

Role of Processed Foods

As I mentioned earlier, processed foods contain less nutrition, more salt, sugar, high fructose corn syrup, hydrogenated oils, preservatives, artificial colors, emulsifiers, artificial flavours, and promote inflammation in our body. Studies have shown that inflammation equals disease. These companies have their bottom line in mind when creating these products and therefore these foods are created with highly-processed ingredients that are often of the lowest and cheapest quality in order to make the highest profit.

According to Dr. Robert Lustig, author of *Metabolical*, "we have learned that sugar (in all its forms), is the main component of processed foods which is the primary driver of four chronic disease (including type 2 diabetes) and likely another five. These diseases total about 75. It's the consumption of refined carbohydrate that's associated with type 2 diabetes". And in a study by JAMA, they found that the higher portion of processed foods in the diet, the higher the risk of type 2 diabetes. Multiple studies have shown a correlation between processed food, sugar consumption, and type 2 diabetes.

In addition, many processed food containers contain both phthalates and bisphenol, which are thought to interfere with our metabolism. Ultra-processed foods have also been associated with insulin resistance, diabetes, abdominal obesity, and hypertension. Plastic packaging and lined cardboard wrapping, as well as canned products can all impact our health by interfering with our hormone balance, with some studies showing they may be related to infertility, hormone-related cancers, and ADHD. By reducing the number of processed foods you eat, you will automatically be reducing your exposure to BPA, phalates, endocrine disruptors, and chemical additives.

But what counts as "processed"? Is it the bag of frozen fruits or peas? Is it the frozen hamburger patties? Is it the can of soup? Is it that cheap box of stove-top stuffing? The box of crackers or cereal? Or maybe the package of instant noodle soup? The answer is yes to all of them. Some processed foods have more additives, while others are a much cleaner option.

Frozen fruit and vegetables contain the product and not much else. They are harvested, washed to remove dirt and pesticides, slightly blanched in boiling water to kill any enzymes, and then flash frozen. These products will have one ingredient on the package and are a cheaper and still a healthy way to get the nutrients we need. Ironically, if you read the directions on the package, it often tells you to add salt and sugar during preparation. Please do not do this.

Frozen fruits and vegetables can be a great option during the winter or if you live in a more remote location. For example, fresh avocadoes are cheap in Mexico but crazy-expensive in Canada, especially in the winter. Frozen avocadoes are cheaper and easily found in the grocery store. Frozen fruits and vegetables can allow us to have a wider variety of foods at a lower price.

The foods you need to be wary of are those with multiple ingredients. These are the food products containing high levels of sugar, salt, preservatives, artificial flavoring, artificial coloring, emulsifiers, and more. These are the packages with the list of ingredients we cannot pronounce or recognize.

Let's look at a popular instant soup mix to understand what a processed food truly is:

"It may contain enriched wheat flour: This is highly-processed flour in which all nutrients were removed during processing, so they have tried to put some back in.

"Palm oil: Saturated fats that raise cholesterol, not to mention palm oil is a major cause of deforestation.

"Salt: Half a package contains 25% of maximum daily sodium requirements and most people eat the whole package.

"Guar gum: Agrochemical from the guar bean which is used as a thickener.

"Garlic powder.

"Artificial chicken: Combination of a hexose, a bland protein hydrolysate and an arachidonic acid compound .

"Cysteine/or Cystine: Or a nontoxic acid addition salt.

"Monosodium Glutamate: MSG has been related to toxicity, metabolic disorders, obesity, and can cause migraines.

"Sugar.

"Yeast extract

"Turmeric powder

"white pepper.

"Disodium Inosinate and Disodium Guanylate: Linked to attention deficit disorder, insomnia, sciatica, and slurred speech.

"Dried leek.

"Caramel: Coloring made from sugar.

"**Wheat:** White highly processed flour.

Does knowing what the ingredients are make you want to purchase this product? No, of course not, but the advertising does.

Ironically, the more processed a food product is, the more you will see it advertised. Companies pay big bucks for these commercials, and we are constantly exposed to them. Think about the commercials you see on television. High-sugar breakfast cereals, cola, fast food restaurants (McDonalds, Burger King, Wendy's), pizza (Dominos, Papa Johns, Pizza Hut), and snack foods (Lays chips, Pringles, Frito, Doritos).

I can still remember the McDonald's jingles from the television ads when I was a child! Now think about how often you see an ad for fresh fruits or vegetables? It is no wonder we are so tempted by processed foods, and why as a society we are getting sicker and fatter. Children are highly susceptible to advertising and companies specifically target children to start their eating and buying habits early in life.

Take foods that have multiple ingredients or those with ingredients you cannot recognize or pronounce out of your diet and focus on eating real food, and foods you prepare yourself. Stop bringing unhealthy foods into your home so that you are not tempted. If you have to put on your coat, drive to the store, and buy your temptation foods, you are less likely to eat it. If you do choose to buy a processed food product, buy it in smaller portion sizes. For example, buy a small individual bag of potato chips instead of the giant family-size bag. Yes, it is cheaper to buy in bulk, but what is the cost to your health?

Have you ever said, "I'm just going to finish up this package because I don't want to waste food"? I know I have! I was raised to finish everything on my plate because "there were starving children in Africa." I'm going to let you in on a little secret. Finishing that package just because you already paid for it isn't going to help your health. In fact, if you finish the product, you are more likely to buy it again because habits kick in and your best intentions will be forgotten. I know some health gurus will tell you to toss all those products into the garbage and start fresh, which works for some people. But if you are like me and feel guilty for wasting money and food (still thinking about those starving children here) your subconscious just won't let you. The guilt will drive you crazy. And you can't donate it because it is already opened, and you don't want to give someone else unhealthy food. And what if you change your mind and want it again? Then you will have wasted the food and the money.

So here is another option, keep the half-eaten package and buy a better, healthier product. Eat the healthier food and see how you feel. Do you feel guilty for wasting money? Well, technically it isn't wasted because the other product is still there. Do you feel happier knowing you made a healthier choice? Do you feel less stressed because your old "go to" comfort food is still there in case you need it?

Basically, I am telling you to do what feels right to you. If the thought of tossing out food makes you feel anxious and stressed, then don't do it. If the thought of keeping unhealthy food in the house makes you feel stressed out, then toss it. If you feel better slowly weaning yourself off unhealthy foods and replacing them with healthier options, then this is the right way to go. Some people are "all or nothing" and need a clean slate. Others need to go more slowly to adjust to change gradually. There is no right or wrong way! There is only the way that works for you.

Action Items:

❖ Avoid television in the evening to avoid food advertising.
❖ Remove processed foods from your home that contain multiple ingredients (especially those you cannot pronounce).
❖ Create a plan to remind yourself of your healthy eating.

Quitting Sugar

When you decide to reduce or eliminate added sugar from your diet, you will need to make a conscious effort, because sugar is added to almost all processed foods, and we are constantly exposed to it. It is added to more foods than you can imagine. Sugar is addictive and can be hard to remove from our diet. The taste releases endorphins in our brain, making us crave more of it. Some people need to wean themselves off slowly while others are a "cold turkey" kind of person. How you choose to reduce and/or remove excess sugar from your diet is up to you.

Now, I am not talking about natural sugars found in fruit or berries, but processed sugar in all its names and forms. The American Heart Association recommends no more than six teaspoons of sugar per day, but the average person has over seventeen; this number is rising every year. To manage type 2 diabetes, we need to eliminate added sugar from our diet.

Added sugar has many names and many of them end in "ose." You need to become familiar with the names so you can recognize them on the ingredients of your packaged food. Sucrose, fructose, lactose, maltose, dextrose, galactose, brown rice sugar, molasses, date sugar, beet sugar, grape sugar, cane sugar, high fructose corn syrup, brown sugar, and agave carob syrup, cane juice crystals, fruit juice concentrate, honey, and sucanat are just a few of the more popular names. There are over fifty-six different names for added sugar! Many processed ingredients have multiple types in the same product, and just because a name sounds natural doesn't mean it is healthy for us.

Many people ask if they can switch to honey because it is more natural, and while raw unprocessed honey does have antifungal, anti-inflammatory properties, it still breaks down into glucose in the body. Save honey for times you have a sore throat and put a tiny bit in a cup of tea, but don't use it as an alternative to sugar.

What about sugar substitutes such as aspartame, sucralose, stevia, Splenda, or xylitol? Are these a better choice than sugar? The short answer is no, they are not better for us. According to a study in the National Library of Medicine, animal studies indicate that artificial sweeteners may cause weight gain, brain tumours, bladder cancer, and can trick our body into producing insulin while not satisfying the craving for sweetness, as it does not produce endorphins in the brain. Because it doesn't satisfy the sweetness, we reach for other foods to fill that need. Some sweeteners cause bloating, diarrhea, gas, or may have a laxative effect in some people, while in others it damages the gut microbiota that keep us healthy. There are reports of mood swings, depression, and panic attacks when people are weaned off artificial sweeteners. Artificial sweeteners created in a laboratory are not the answer. If you are an insulin dependent diabetic, then a tiny amount of artificial sweetener such as stevia may allow you to have a wider variety of foods. However it is my opinion that artificial sweeteners carry too much risk and that focusing on the most natural foods is better for our body.

For those weaning themselves off added sugar slowly, you can try having smaller portions of sugary food. For example, instead of a whole chocolate bar, have one piece. This may be enough to satisfy the craving. You can also try combining it with a more nutritious food or fibre to slow the absorption of the glucose. For example, having a banana with ice cream. Or reaching for sweet fruits instead of processed sugar foods. This will still provide the sweetness you are craving, but with fibre and nutrition.

If you are craving a particular food, don't shop around eating multiple things in the kitchen trying to fill that craving. You may end up eating hundreds of calories because nothing else other than that food stops the craving. Have a small portion, preferably combined with a more nutritious one, and satisfy the craving.

If you are a "cold turkey" kind of person, then the first seventy-two hours may be a bit tough. During this period, I suggest chewing mint gum, brushing your teeth (the minty flavour is strong enough to stop many cravings), go for a walk or other exercise, or have a change of scenery to take your mind off the craving. Keep yourself hydrated by drinking plain or flavored water.

Regardless of which method you choose, be sure to eat regularly so you do not have excess hunger pushing you toward your sugar craving. When we are over-hungry it is easy to eat anything in sight until the pain of hunger passes. Drink plenty of water to help flush out your system and keep your hands busy. Keeping our hands busy keeps us from snacking mindlessly. You might choose to do your nails, knit, or crochet, play scrabble, draw, work in your garden, build model airplanes, or play with a fidget toy. I had one client who started knitting while watching television to stop herself from eating sugary foods. Not only did she kick the sugar habit and drop twenty pounds, but she is now selling beautiful, knitted blankets.

Additionally, be sure to get a good night's sleep, as we all make poor food choices when we are tired. Scientists have discovered that a lack of sleep stimulates the hormone "ghrelin," which tells our brain that we are hungry. Then, our brain enhances the olfaction capacity meaning we reach for foods with certain smells. This is why you want pizza instead of a spinach salad. Combine this with our craving for more energy, and we are reaching for unhealthy foods.

Keep a healthy snack in your bag for those afternoon pick-me-ups instead of heading for the vending machine or the local Starbucks. Breaking old eating habits that may trigger a sugar craving is really important. For example, if you always have a muffin with coffee at your local café, you may want to avoid the location or choose a different drink.

Food, drinks, and location can all be craving triggers. This is why you will see people who don't smoke have a cigarette when they are drinking alcohol. In the past, alcohol and cigarettes went together and the craving was activated if one product or the other was reintroduced. Because we are creatures of habit, we need to create new habits to replace old ones. If there are muffins or other pastries at your morning work meetings, offer to bring in a healthier option such as fruit or chew gum so you won't eat the muffins.

Make an effort to reduce your stress. When we face a stressful situation, our body releases cortisol, our stress hormone, which prepares the body for a fight or flight situation. It does this by flooding the body with glucose for immediate energy to our large muscles and stops insulin production so that glucose can't be stored. Cortisol narrows the arteries and epinephrine increases our heart-rate, making our blood pump harder. Once the situation is resolved, our hormone levels return to normal. The problem lies in constant stress and increased cortisol levels, which consistently lead to higher glucose levels, and therefore increased sugar.

When we are happy, joyful, and energetic we do not produce the same level of cortisol, nor do we have the same psychological need for sugary foods. But when we are tired, angry, bored, or unfulfilled we have a need to fill that empty space in our life. Create a life that is fulfilling, whether it is through your family, job, volunteer work, or hobbies. Incorporate activities that bring you joy and produce natural endorphins. Take the time to reduce the mental and emotional stress in your life with the tips mentioned in this book.

They say that drinking apple cider vinegar in water throughout the day helps to keep sugar cravings at bay. I have never tried this personally (because I do not like the taste of apple cider vinegar) but it might just work for you. I have found that lemon water (hot or cold) works very well for me and is much easier to obtain at restaurants than apple cider vinegar.

You can also try giving yourself a flavor that is not sweet. For example, try a bitter food when craving a sweet food, as this can stop the craving. Training yourself to like more bitter foods, such as fermented foods or unsweetened dark chocolate, can help remove sweetness cravings.

Remember that you are not "bad" if you have a sugar-sweetened food. You are not your food choices. You will have good days and you will have days when the sugar craving wins. Take each day at a time and try to make the best choices you can in the moment. Be kind to yourself and remember that sugar is an addiction and can take time and effort to overcome.

There are some amino acids such as GABA, Tyrosine, and Tryptophan that may help with intense sugar cravings. If you are a stress eater, taking GABA may help to eliminate these cravings by making you feel more relaxed. Tryptophan helps to address the low-serotonin sugar cravings that normally happen late-afternoon or in the evening, or when we are comfort-eating to make ourselves feel better. If you are tired and eating for energy, then tyrosine may help you to feel more energetic. Many people find that taking amino acids helps in reducing sugar cravings as well as cravings for processed carbohydrates.

I explain the pros and cons of amino acids a little later in the book, as well as the importance of working with your doctor or a nutritionist like myself before self-prescribing amino acids. While amino acids are found naturally in foods, supplemental amino acids can interact with many medications, so talk to your doctor or pharmacist before you start taking them.

Action Items:

- ❖ Choose how you will wean yourself off sugar.
- ❖ Make a plan to remind yourself.
- ❖ How will you keep your hands busy?
- ❖ Get a good night's sleep.
- ❖ Buy healthy snacks for home and work.

The Ketogenic Diet

There are many versions of the ketogenic diet on social media today: cyclical, high protein, standard, targeted, and dirty keto. The basis of a ketogenic diet is that when we drop our carbohydrate intake to a very low amount, but retain a high fat intake, we force the body to produce ketones in the liver and burn fats for energy rather than using glucose.

The idea is that by removing most of the glucose from the diet it drastically reduces the amount of insulin produced, allowing the person to lose weight and reduce blood pressure, prediabetes, type 2 diabetes, and metabolic syndrome. Studies have also shown the keto diet is helpful for slowing the progression of Alzheimer's, dementia, Parkinson's, and can be beneficial for those with epilepsy and polycystic ovary syndrome.

The downside of a long-term keto is the lack of the fibre, vitamins, and minerals that carbohydrates provide which may have a negative effect on some people. Additionally, many people eat too much saturated fat when making up the carbohydrates missing in their diet, which can cause heart disease, high blood pressure, poor cholesterol levels, and some types of cancers. It is also a very restrictive eating program that many find difficult to follow.

The keto diet should never be followed by a pregnant woman as there is a higher risk of neural tube defects (defects in the brain, spine, or spinal cord) in the baby. If you are losing weight and trying to get pregnant, I also strongly advise against a keto diet as you will not get the vitamins, minerals, and phytonutrients the baby needs to develop properly should you get pregnant.

Another downside to keto is the risk of kidney stones and kidney damage due to the high uric acid levels. While there are some people who do very well on these types of strict diets, the majority of people are more successful on a balanced dietary plan that is less restrictive and has fewer risks.

If you have a large amount of weight to lose, have very high blood glucose levels, or choose to follow a ketogenic diet after consultation with your doctor, it is important to understand the difference between the "keto diets" you find online that include massive amounts of unhealthy fats, and the true ketogenic healthy diet.

The healthy keto diet I am talking about contains higher amounts of healthy fats, such as cold-water fish, nuts, seeds, olives, olive oil, and avocados. It does not include putting butter in your coffee or huge amounts of bacon and other animal fats. A healthy keto diet includes lean protein such as chicken breast, turkey, pork, lean cuts of beef, and fish. Be sure your sources of lean protein are grass-fed, non-hormone, organic sources to avoid any toxins or high omega-6 fatty acids. Non-starchy vegetables grown above the ground are consumed to ensure adequate fibre, mineral, and vitamin intake. These will include peppers, cucumbers, leafy greens, celery, radish, broccoli, Brussel sprouts, cabbage, asparagus, eggplant, zucchini, tomatoes, green beans, and cauliflower. Vegetables grown in the ground such as potatoes, carrots, beets, etc. are higher in carbohydrates and should be avoided on this diet or eaten in very small amounts. Please note that medications such as Warfarin, Coumadin, or Jantoven may be impacted by eating more vegetables than usual containing a high amount of vitamin K. Talk to your doctor before starting any new diet and explain the foods you will be eating.

On a strict ketogenic diet only 5 to 10% of your diet is made up of healthy carbohydrates and, depending on your weight and calorie intake, this may equate to approximately twenty grams. It is important to track your food using an online food counter such as Chronometer, Carb Manager, or My Fitness App.

Grains and high-starch vegetables such as peas and corn are extremely limited because they are high in carbohydrates. All processed carbohydrates made from grains are also removed. This will include pasta, baked goods, cereals, and anything including high fructose corn syrup.

Protein intake is 25 to 35% of your dietary intake. Remember, this is lean protein not fatty cuts of meat or processed meats that will drive up your triglyceride levels (we want to keep your heart and liver healthy).

Fat intake will be approximately 60 to 75% of your dietary intake. This may sound like a lot but remember that fat has nine calories per gram whereas carbohydrates and protein have four, so the amount of fat consumed will be much less. Many healthy foods such as meat, eggs, avocados, olives, nuts, seeds, and cold-water fish have a higher amount of healthy fats. You will also be eating small amounts of butter, coconut, and cheese, which adds flavor to your food. Avoid all trans-fat and any product that includes hydrogenated fats. Extra virgin olive oil and avocado oil are great for creating homemade salad dressing and for cooking.

Eating fats will help to absorb fat-soluble vitamins such as A, E, D, and K as well as helping keep our cell membranes (the outer part of our cells) healthy. Our skin, hair, eyes, muscles, and hormone production all depend on fat. It may feel counterintuitive to eat more fat but think of it this way, we feed animals grains (carbohydrates) to fatten them up, and they affect humans the same way. The idea of eating more grains and more carbohydrates to lose weight and lower blood glucose levels just doesn't make sense.

You will be eating protein and fat with every meal in order to reduce the absorption of glucose and keep insulin levels lower. For your body to create ketones, you must stick with the ratios described above to ensure your carbohydrate percentage does not increase. Some people use ketone testing strips to test their urine to ensure that they are in ketosis. These are available online and in most pharmacies.

While some people have lost weight and reduced their blood sugar on this program, you need to decide if it is right for you. You may wish to try this for a short period, such as thirty or sixty days, and rotate between this and the low glycemic carbohydrate program to ensure you are obtaining enough vitamins and minerals to maintain optimal health.

Low Glycemic Carbohydrate Diet

In the Standard American Diet, our carbohydrate levels may be 50 to 60% of our dietary intake. This includes high amounts of grains (in the form of breads, cereal, baked goods, rice, quinoa, and oats) as well as vegetables (including high starch and high glycemic vegetables), fruits, and berries. The old recommendations of nine to twelve servings of these foods were based on the idea that if we lowered our fat intake, we would lose fat. Sadly, this advice gave rise to the large obesity and diabetes epidemic we see today.

The low glycemic carbohydrate dietary plan calls for about 30% of our diet in the form of healthy carbohydrates. If you are following a calorie-controlled plan this would be around ninety grams for a 1,200-calorie meal or one-hundred-and-twelve for a 1,500-calorie meal. Please keep in mind that these are just estimates as your needs are determined by your age, physical activity, weight, and blood sugar control.

We need approximately 100 calories for each pound in order to maintain basic functions. For example, if you weight 150 lbs you need 1500 calories to function. Severe caloric restriction will not help you lose weight as it will slow your metabolism and should never be done without the supervision of your physician. Multiple studies have shown that eating a healthy diet with the proper number of calories will help reduce weight and keep it off.

Whole fruit, leafy greens, vegetables, berries, and a small number of natural grains should be the focus of our carbohydrate intake. Eliminating highly-processed forms of carbohydrates is key. Keep in mind the more processed a carbohydrate is, the higher the sugar (glucose) and the lower the nutritional value. By eliminating these types of foods, you will keep your blood glucose lower, eat more fibre (which slows the absorption of glucose and rise in insulin), and obtain and absorb more nutrients to manage your type 2 diabetes. If you have a large amount of weight to lose, reduce your carbohydrates to 25%, and eat 45% lean healthy proteins and 30% healthy fats.

To calculate your grams of carbohydrates, follow this easy method. Total calories per day multiplied by percentage of carbohydrates divided by four grams.

For example:

1,500 calories x 30% = 450.
450/4 calories per gram = 112 grams of carbohydrates.

Be aware that your doctor may recommend a lower rate of carbohydrate consumption to start.

We are going to focus on eating the low/medium glycemic vegetables, leafy greens, fruits, berries, and melons. Eat one serving per day of whole fruit or berries, and five to seven servings of fresh vegetables. If you need to reduce calories, reduce your serving of vegetables by one serving per day. Complex carbohydrates that are lower glycemic foods absorb and are digested more slowly, which causes a slower and smaller rise in blood sugar levels and keeps you feeling full longer. If you suffer from constipation, eat two servings of whole fruit or berries and five to six servings of vegetables. If you do not have access to fresh vegetables, frozen is your next best option. Avoid canned fruits and vegetables, as the processing removes most of the fibre and nutrition and canned fruit is high in sugar and salt.

I know you probably have your favourite fruits and vegetables that are you "go to" when you get groceries, but it is time to change things up. Be sure to eat a variety of foods in order to get the maximum variety of vitamins, minerals, and phytonutrients because different foods have different levels of nutrients. Try to eat an orange vegetable such as carrots, squash, peppers, sweet potato, and pumpkin at least twice a week, as these contain vitamin A, which most people are deficient in. Try different types of leafy greens, different fruits, vegetables, berries, and melons. Did you know that there are over 7,500 varieties of apple grown around the world? How many have you tried? By expanding our food repertoire, we can avoid food boredom and enhance our nutritional intake.

Aim to eat two cups of leafy greens daily (in addition to your vegetables) and try to mix up the type of leafy greens you eat as they don't all provide the exact amount of nutrients. Some great ways to eat leafy greens are in salads, wraps, green smoothies, on sandwiches, or in a stir fry.

Eat only one serving of processed grains per day or none if you can avoid them. One serving is one piece of bread, half a bagel, a small roll, or 3/4 cup of pasta. I know this may seem a bit of a challenge, after all we are accustomed to eating large portions of processed grains in our diets. Cereal for breakfast, a sandwich for lunch, and pasta for dinner, plus a cookie or muffin during the day. Finding alternative meals does take a bit of planning in the beginning but cutting out processed grains has a huge impact on our insulin levels, weight, digestive health, energy, and overall health.

Try having oatmeal with berries, or scrambled eggs with spinach for breakfast. You could also try soup, or a salad with protein at lunch, and a lean protein with vegetables for dinner. Start by changing one meal, then change another, and then the final one. You may find that changing dinner first is easier for you, as it is the time when most members of the family are at home. You decide which meal you want to address first and make the necessary changes.

Eat one to two servings of unprocessed grains such as brown rice, quinoa, millet, or spelt a day (dependent upon weight and weight-loss goals). If you need to lower calories to lose weight, reduce from two servings to one per day as these are more caloric than vegetables. If you find that grains cause bloating or fatigue, remove any grains that contain gluten.

40% of daily calories should be from lean protein, whether that is from animal protein or vegetarian sources. This is equivalent to three servings of lean protein a day. A serving size is the size of a deck of cards or 3/4 of a cup of vegetarian sources (such as tofu or lentils) or two eggs. Be aware that serving sizes in restaurants are often twice the amount or more of a single serving.

Protein will help keep you feeling full longer, and we need it to build muscles and aid brain function and healing.

Additionally, it can help to slow the absorption of glucose, helping to stabilize our blood glucose and insulin levels (remember we want to keep our insulin levels low and steady). If you are following a calorie-counting plan, 1,200 calories would be approximately one-hundred-and-twenty grams of protein, or one-hundred-and-fifty grams on a 1,500-calorie plan. Just like with carbohydrates, the type of protein we consume is important and excess protein will be stored as adipose tissue.

You will be consuming 30% of your food as healthy fats which lower the glycemic load of our food as well as providing us the building blocks for needed hormones and cell growth. If you are following a calorie-counting plan, 1,200 calories means approximately forty grams of fat, and a 1,500-calorie plan would be sixty-six grams. Excessive poor quality fat intake is a major factor in high blood pressure, heart disease, obesity, and colon cancer so be sure to consume only healthy fats and try stay to the 30% ratio. Healthy fats include olives, avocado, nuts, seeds (such as almonds, walnuts, cashews, pumpkin seeds, sunflower seeds, flax seeds, and chia seeds), cold-water fish, and eggs.

Many foods are counted as both a protein and a fat which gets a bit confusing. Meat, fish, nuts, seeds, dairy, and beans contain both protein and fats. This is why an online food tracker is helpful.

Intermittent Fasting

Intermittent fasting (IF) is the practice of restricting eating within certain hours. I am not recommending an extreme IF practice (such as eating all your daily calories within a two-hour window) as this can cause our cortisol levels to rise, create food cravings and binge eating. Not to mention who wants to feel hungry all day long?

According to Dr. Robert H. Lustig, "by depriving your liver of calories for fourteen to sixteen hours per day, IF gives it a chance to activate AMP-kinase, supress mTOR, increase autophagy, chew up some of the liver fat that's been stored, improve insulin resistance and lower your insulin." Studies have shown intermittent fasting helps lower the risk of type 2 diabetes by improving glucose control, aiding in weight loss, protecting brain and cardiovascular function, reducing inflammation, improving memory, and by helping improve digestion.

An article in PubMed stated the majority of available research demonstrates intermittent fasting is effective at reducing body weight, decreasing fasting glucose, decreasing fasting insulin, reducing insulin resistance, decreasing levels of leptin, and increasing levels of adiponectin. In addition, some studies found patients were able to reverse their need for insulin therapy during therapeutic intermittent fasting protocols (please only do this under the supervision of your doctor).

Because you are still eating throughout your busy day, there is no feeling of "starvation" or deprivation that may lead to binging. IF can promote a better relationship with food as food is not seen as "the enemy" but as the nutrition that feeds our body and keeps us strong and healthy.

For the reasons mentioned above, we are going to start with a ten-hour IF program. This means you have ten hours to consume all your meals in a day, followed by fourteen hours with no food. From the time you eat breakfast, count ten hours forward, and your last meal must be completed by this time. Once you find the ten-hour window easy, you can switch to an eight-hour eating window with sixteen hours with no food. Do this gradually by reducing an hour at a time. Our bodies need a continual intake of food throughout our busy days, so do not go below the eight-hour eating window as this can cause stress on our body, slow our metabolism and cause weight gain.

If you are constantly thinking about food, or the idea of restricting your eating time causes you anxiety, you may not be mentally ready for an eight-hour intermittent fasting program. Do what feels right for you. When you are ready, gradually move from the ten-hour window to an eight-hour window. You should not feel stressed, anxious, be constantly thinking about food, or wanting to binge-eat during this process. If you start to feel anxious, simply return to the ten-hour window, and when you are ready, start again.

By keeping our food consumption within a specific window, our body is allowed fourteen hours or more with no food consumption, meaning there is no insulin production. It also allows our body to use our fat stores as an energy source. Intermittent fasting can reduce levels of fasting insulin and glucose, assist in weight loss, and help to control our eating habits.

When you are not eating, you are allowed water, unsweetened green, herbal, or spearmint tea (may help reduce androgens for those with PCOS), or red raspberry leaf tea (may help reduce estrogen for those who are estrogen-dominant). It is important to stay hydrated, which helps us to ensure proper elimination, avoid constipation, and balance our blood pressure. Dehydration also causes fatigue, which can make us think we are hungry and want to reach for sugary foods for energy. Avoid more than one cup of caffeinated tea or coffee, and only drink caffeine in the morning so it does not interfere with your sleep.

Have your last meal two hours before bedtime, then sleep eight to ten hours. Not eating right before bed can also assist in reducing bloating, indigestion, and heart burn. If drinking fluids keeps you up at night, stop all fluids with your last meal. We want you to have a deep and refreshing sleep without having to wake to use the washroom. Be sure you do not overeat during the feasting hours and focus on whole nutritious foods in the proper portion sizes. Stick to eating low glycemic foods with plenty of fiber in your correct number of portions.

While the majority of research shows that intermittent fasting can assist in weight loss, decrease fasting glucose, decrease fasting insulin, reduce insulin resistance, and decrease levels of leptin, women who are pregnant, insulin dependent diabetic, or those with eating disorders should never practice intermittent fasting without consulting their doctor first. If you are an insulin dependent diabetic, following a keto diet and using intermittent fasting can lead to a dangerous condition known as diabetic ketoacidosis. Always discuss with your doctor before beginning any dietary program.

Action Plan:

- ❖ Decide what you will drink in your non-eating hours.
- ❖ Purchase any teas or lemons you require.
- ❖ Decide how you will avoid eating in the evening and implement your reminders.

Exercise

A sedentary lifestyle is a known contributor to the increase in type 2 diabetes. We sit in our daily commute, then sit in an office all day. In the evening we watch television or play games on our computers. We do not even need to go shopping or out for food as our groceries and meals are delivered to our doorstep. Physical education programs at some schools are being removed from the curriculum due to the cost, and there are not always safe areas in some neighborhoods for play. Our children are constantly on their phones, computers, or sitting in front of the television. We have become a generation of sitters.

Adults need thirty minutes of exercise a day a week to maintain their current weight. If you are overweight you may need to add to this level, depending on the type of exercise you do, your current activity level, and the amount of weight you need to lose. Children over six years of age need an hour a day of moderate to vigorous aerobic activity.

Please understand that this does not mean that the exercise must all be done at the same time. Dividing the exercise time throughout the day can have many health benefits and make it easier to fit into a busy day. For example, your child may walk to and from school for fifteen minutes, play basketball for thirty minutes after school, and walk the dog for fifteen minutes in the evening.

Regular exercise can manage the symptoms of type 2 diabetes as it improves insulin sensitivity, reduces blood sugar levels, reduces inflammation in the body, and also improves blood pressure and lipid profiles (cholesterol and triglycerides). Exercise also reduces the risk of heart disease and regulates body weight by reducing body fat percentage and enhancing lean muscle. Be sure to consult your doctor before beginning any exercise program to ensure you do not have hypertension or other health issues that may affect your performance.

While aerobic exercise is good for overall weight loss, I have found that long steady-state cardio best increases cortisol and, in turn, increases insulin levels. The best form of exercise is high intensity interval training (HIIT) for a shorter period. Not only will this keep your cortisol levels lower, but it can be completed in half the time which is perfect for people who are busy.

Studies show that HIIT is good for type 2 diabetes, non-alcoholic fatty liver disease, heart disease, and high cholesterol. HIIT involves several minutes of high intensity followed by a minute of low intensity. For example, you may walk on a high incline for three minutes then lower to zero incline for one. From there, gradually build up the amount of time your body is under stress. High intensity interval training is only done for up to fifteen minutes followed by a cool down and gentle stretching.

Whether you choose to use a stationary bicycle, treadmill, elliptical trainer, or jogging, it doesn't really matter. I recommend you mix it up to avoid boredom and to get the best of each of these exercises. Start with one minute of intense exercise (as hard as you can), then slow for a minute, then repeat. Gradually build up the time you are doing intense exercise to five minutes before you have your lower-level minute. If you are obese you may need to start at a lower intensity and build your way up.

The key to HIIT is the intensity. If you are chatting with the person next to you then you are not working hard enough. You should be panting, only able to get out a few words with some effort. If you cannot speak at all, you are working too hard and need to reduce the intensity. Another option for those who need a more gradual approach is to do a fifteen- to thirty-second interval at 80% intensity followed by two to three minutes of lower intensity. Gradually build up the intensity until you are close to 100%, then begin to increase the time of your higher level. Go slowly so that you do not injure yourself.

I also want you to try flexibility exercises such as stretching, tai chi, or yoga. Flexibility exercises improve blood circulation and muscles in areas that support our posture and movement, therefore decreasing the pressure on our spine and core muscles over time. These exercises help to relieve back pain and prevent injuries and balance issues. As we age our muscles lose their elasticity, strength, and mobility which makes it easier to become injured. If you have ever slipped on ice and jarred your back, you will understand the need for flexibility in your body.

Yoga and tai chi are also great for improving breathing, relaxing the body and mind, and therefore relieving stress. According to a 2018 study in the Journal of Endocrinology and Metabolism, yoga increases the number of insulin receptors, reduces fasting insulin levels, and helps to normalize the insulin-to-glucose ratio. The wonderful thing about yoga is it can be done anywhere, at home, at a yoga studio, or even in a hotel room.

The next type of exercise I want you to perform is a weightlifting or resistance exercise. There are a couple of reasons why this type of exercise is important. First, resistance exercise helps to build stronger bones. Bone must be exposed to a mechanical load (weight) in order to increase in density and strength. I'm sure that you have seen an older woman who appeared frail and bent over? Or know of someone who has fallen and broken her hip and had a long recovery period? This is due to a lack of bone density. It takes approximately four months of weight-bearing exercises to build up bone density. Our bones are constantly being broken down to provide us with calcium for regulating our heartbeat, helping muscles contract, and for nerve function and blood clotting, and are then regrown when we ingest calcium. Weight-bearing exercises need to be done throughout our lifetime.

Weight training also allows us to reshape the body, which can provide greater self-esteem. Perhaps you wish to build your booty? Or reshape the shoulders? Or lose the jiggle on the back of your arms? Weightlifting is the way to do these things. By working on specific body parts each time you exercise, you can complete your workout in a shorter period of time. Increased muscle mass also burns more calories at rest. And who doesn't want that? Don't worry, you won't look like a body builder with huge manly muscles! It takes women years of training, and a very specific program, to build muscles up to that size. Weight training will give you the sexy sculpted look with strong bones and additional strength.

Another option is to use resistance bands, which can be purchased online, or at department stores or pharmacies. Resistance bands are made at different tensile strengths and are a great tool for beginners, the elderly, or for use while travelling. There are many wonderful YouTube videos and books available on resistance band exercises.

You should aim to work out five days per week. Alternate your HIIT days and weightlifting / resistance band days with a day of flexibility training in between. For example: Monday HIIT, Tuesday Yoga, Wednesday weightlifting, Thursday rest day, Friday HIIT, Saturday Yoga, Sunday weightlifting. You can switch up the type of HIIT and flexibility exercise to avoid getting bored. Your rest day is important so be sure to take it. It doesn't mean you can't move but give your body a break. Our body creates muscle by first breaking down the muscle with microscopic tears, which then heal make the muscle stronger than it was before. Rest days are important for healing.

Before you begin any exercise program, consult your doctor to ensure it is safe, as well as a certified trainer to ensure you have proper form during weight training. It is easy to hurt yourself and an injury can set you back weeks. Many gyms will provide an orientation, or you can hire a personal trainer for a few sessions to get you started. Begin with a low weight to learn the correct form and build up gradually. Be sure to do exercises for both sides of the muscle to prevent a weakness on the other side. For example, if you are exercising your abdominal muscles, be sure to exercise your back muscles as well for strength and a well-proportioned look. Always ease into an exercise routine and build up slowly.

Blood sugar levels can be impacted by exercise and will vary depending on the type and length of exercise, whether you are insulin dependent, your age, weight, and level of fitness. Blood sugar typically rises during the exercise because our body is compensating for the additional stress we are placing on it. Heavy weightlifting, competitive sports, endurance sports, and intense workouts can raise adrenaline, which stimulates our liver to release glucose.

If you are using a blood glucose monitor, check your levels before and after exercise to see how your body reacts to the different types of exercise you perform. If you take insulin, you may be at a risk of hypoglycemia (low blood sugar) after strenuous exercise and should take precautions. Tell your coach or workout buddy that you are diabetic just in case there is an issue, and/or wear a diabetes bracelet so you can receive the help you need if you are unable to communicate. If you do suffer from hypoglycemia, you may find that eating a small snack before and after your workout is helpful.

If you suffer from high cholesterol and take statins, you may find that your joints or muscles ache and doing high impact workouts may be more difficult. Statins can also increase the risk of damaging your joints during intense workouts. You may find that lowering the intensity of your workout helps. You could also switch to balance and stretching exercises (such as yoga or tai chi) or warm the joints and muscles through a sauna or massage, for example, to help your body feel more limber.

Some high blood pressure medications, such as beta blockers, will slow your heart rate which means you may not reach your target heart rate. Your blood pressure may be impacted for several hours after exercise (especially long session cardio) which may require an adjustment to medication. Be sure to talk to your doctor about your exercise program to determine if you need a change in medication or whether you should take your medication or exercise at a different time of the day.

Some of you may be saying that you don't have time to exercise because you are too busy. But if you don't make time for health, you will make time for illness. There is always a way to fit exercise into our day and I challenge you to try to add in as many ways as you can. Perhaps you do not have the luxury of a gym membership or home equipment? Not a problem! Here are some ways to exercise at no cost.

The squat challenge is an easy one and can be done at home or in any public bathroom. Start day one with ten squats and add ten each day until you get to one hundred squats. Mix up the type of squats you do to avoid boredom and get better exercise. Did you know there are forty-five different types of squats? You can split the squats up during the day by doing some first thing in the morning and the rest in the evening. You can do simple squats in any bathroom stall or at your desk at work. You can do squats in a hotel room or in a park. Squats are great for the legs, and if you do enough of them in a row you will get your heart rate up.

Walking is great exercise and all you need is a pair of shoes! You can do it anywhere, anytime, alone or with a friend. To raise the intensity, try walking up hills or on a beach. There are many people who walk through malls early in the morning before they open to walk during bad weather or to ensure their safety.

Want to boost your endurance? Try stair climbing! You don't need to go to a gym just use the staircase at work, a mall, or any public building. Stair climbing is a great cardiovascular workout, and it is fabulous for the legs and booty.

There are many free online workouts on YouTube you can follow that are available for all fitness levels. Whether you are looking for an exercise program using your own bodyweight as resistance or want to learn to do yoga—there is something for everyone.

Action Items:

- ❖ Get doctor's approval before beginning. Have cholesterol levels, glucose, and blood pressure checked.
- ❖ Choose your types of exercise.
- ❖ How will you remind yourself to exercise?

Stress and our Health

We all experience stress at one time or another; there is no getting away from it. Whether it is from home, work, family, friends, the weather, or current events—stress is part of our everyday lives. Turn on the news and all we hear is negativity. Our phones send us constant updates on world conflicts and events. We are overloaded with constant negativity, bad news and conflict. There is no getting away from stress, but *how* we deal with it is the key to better health. This is the difference between good health and poor health both physically and mentally. While "stress" is not considered a medical illness in itself it can still have a huge impact on our body, and we need to learn to deal with it effectively.

When we are confronted with a stressful situation or event, our body first releases adrenaline (which helps us jump out of the way of a car, or run from a vicious dog), and then our adrenal glands pump out cortisol to lower the adrenaline and provide us with long-lasting strength and stamina. Cortisol is the hormone that allows us to deal with ongoing physical, emotional, or mental stress such as an illness, army boot camp, a horrible boss, etc.

The problems arise when constant stress in our life causes continual release of adrenaline and cortisol, leaving us feeling worn out and unable to function properly. Chronic stress and high levels of cortisol interfere with our ability to use insulin effectively. Now you might be thinking that you don't have that much stress in your life, so this doesn't affect you. It is important to understand our body reacts the same whether it is a physical threat, high sugar / low protein food, caffeine, chronic infection, exposure to chemicals, or long-term illness. Chronic stress can wear out our adrenal glands, creating an inability to create cortisol to cope, which can lead to physical problems such as poor immunity, heart disease, obesity, and damaged brain cells.

Chronic stress, regardless of whether it's from high sugar consumption or intense situations, has a huge impact on our body and can produce symptoms such as fatigue, irritability, headaches, intestinal issues (constipation, bloating, or diarrhea), anxiety, depression, weight gain, increased blood pressure, poor sleep, and interfere with our menstrual cycle. An elevated stress hormone supresses the thyroid, and our immune function. Decreased thyroid function slows down the liver detoxification process (remember, the thyroid determines the speed of our metabolism), and as the liver detox slows, gut function declines which prevents toxins, chemicals, and extra estrogen from being processed out of the body.

This slow liver detoxification can cause SIBO (small intestinal bacteria overgrowth), leaky gut, and estrogen dominance. As our gut function declines, hormone imbalances increase, which can contribute to insulin and leptin resistance. When our adrenal system can no longer cope, we get the feeling of "I can't take anymore." This is the tipping point for many people, when our mental, and emotional stress manifests in our body and we feel overwhelmed, sick, and exhausted.

Try reducing stress factors in your life by avoiding toxic people or by changing your work or home environment. It's okay to set boundaries and not allow negative or toxic people in your life. While it may seem "mean" to set boundaries or remove these people, I promise you will feel much better after. When I finally removed the toxic people in my life, it was as if a weight had been lifted off my shoulders. At first, I felt guilty, but then I came to the realization that I am not responsible for how someone else feels or acts and that I need to take care of myself first. Other things I realized are that it is okay not to talk to the cranky person at work every morning, and that it is not my responsibility to cheer people up nor to listen to negative rants on a daily basis. I started taking my lunch breaks and using them to go for a walk away from the office or sit in my car on rainy days, listening to peaceful music, instead of working through them. I learned to protect my own mental wellbeing, which in turn created for myself a much better physical, mental, and emotional state.

Other stress factors may be caring for children or elderly parents. Ask others for help! They say it takes a village to raise a child, and I believe this. Getting a friend or family member to provide babysitting or taking your unwell parent out for a few hours (or staying in to sit with them if required) can be a huge mental health break. You do not have to be Super Woman/Man. There is no weakness in asking for help. If you are caring for a parent, there are organizations that may be able to provide respite care, giving you a much-needed break.

Take a "me day" at least once a month. This is a day, or even just a few hours, where you can spend time doing something that is just for you. No shopping for the kids or using the time to clean your house or run errands, this is time spent giving yourself some self-love. Maybe you can go to the movies? Have lunch with a good friend? Have a bubble bath without anyone banging on the door or screaming in the hallway? Get your nails done? Wander around a bookstore? It doesn't matter what you do as long as you feel relaxed and happy doing it.

When my daughter was young, I started insisting on a "me" day once a month; to be honest, sometimes I had to fight for it, but I truly believe it saved my sanity. It gave me time to rejuvenate and relax, which made me a happier healthier person. When I tell my clients to take a *me day*, I always get the same look of disbelief. But every single time they come back and tell me the same thing, "Oh my god! I didn't realize how much I needed a few hours to myself. I feel like a new person!"

Reduce the amount of television you and your family watch, as well as video game and cell phone use, especially in the evening. An interesting study by the Journal of Family and Community Medicine showed that the more hours a teenager spends on their cell phone, the higher the rates of anxiety and depression. We are constantly bombarded by noise, electronic lights, advertising, unrealistic social media expectations, and as a result we are over-stimulated, anxious, and have poor-quality sleep. Turn off your electronics when you get home and resist the urge to constantly check your social media. Give yourself a break! Go for a walk, call a friend, or loved one, get outside and play, go to the gym, work in your garden, or read a book.

If traffic stresses you out, try taking a different route to work or leaving earlier. Play happy music that brings you joy and sing in the car. It's okay if you can't sing because this is all about you. Take the train, bus, or carpool to work if that is an option for you, but maybe don't sing on these. Learn and practice deep breathing exercises during traffic jams and be forgiving when someone cuts you off instead of getting angry.

If the clutter in your home causes issues, try embracing minimalism. Personally, having a lot of clutter or things around me creates a lot of anxiety and I can't relax or focus on my work. By cleaning or organizing my environment I feel as though I have taken control and am able to create a more relaxed and stress-free room. Once a year I go through my closet and dresser to remove clothing that no longer fits, or I don't use. I toss out items in my home that are broken and donate what no longer adds value to my life. Because I hate dusting, I don't have lots of little things all over bookshelves or tabletops. The clean look of the space provides me with a feeling of calmness. I get satisfaction in having a clean, tidy, organized space.

If you feel overloaded at work, try delegating to an assistant or talking to your boss about reprioritizing the due dates. Career workload or boredom at work consistently ranks in the top ten stressors. Too much work, a terrible boss, a toxic work environment, or feeling unsatisfied with the work you perform are the most common complaints I hear.

Try meditation to reduce stress or anxiety levels or improve feelings of joy (there are free guided meditations on YouTube), or deep breathing, walking in nature, playing with a pet, a good night's sleep, a vacation, or drinking water.

Now, I'm not suggesting you quit your job, leave your family, and move to a hut on an island—but evaluate what causes you the most stress and determine what you can change to alleviate it. Stress is inevitable but learning to deal with it effectively can make a huge difference in our mental, physical, emotional health and allow our body to use insulin more effectively.

Consider what changes you will make in your life to reduce stress. Use your journal to make a list of everything that stresses you on one side of a piece of paper, no matter how big or small. Then think of some ways you can eliminate or reduce the stress of each item and list them on the opposite side of the paper. Keep an open mind. Often, because we have done something the same way for years, we think we can't make a change, but other options are always available. You could even ask for suggestions from a trusted friend or family member. Write down as many ideas as you can think of, even if they seem far-fetched or impossible. Often, the best idea is the third or fourth one.

Action Items:

- ❖ Identify the stressors in your life and options to deal with them.
- ❖ Book your "me" day for the month and don't cancel on yourself!
- ❖ Reduce screen time and find another activity.
- ❖ Find meditations, stress relief, or deep breathing exercises on YouTube that you enjoy.

Environmental Toxins

While the world was locked down for Covid-19, air pollution dropped significantly, and the animal kingdom began to thrive. Without the impact of humanity on the planet it began to heal. We read articles in the news about pollution, toxins, and pesticides but sadly unless the issues are in our own back yard, we don't really understand the impact they have on our health and how we need to heal our body.

What if I told you that you that you are exposed to over 80,000 chemicals a day? That plastic bottled water containers can leach 24,000 chemicals in our body. That new cars contain two-hundred-and-seventy-five chemicals linked to birth defects, cancer, liver damage and learning impairment. And that there are over 12,000 personal care products that are defined as carcinogens, toxins, or hormone disruptors. Would you be concerned then? According to the NRDC (National Resources Defence Council), "over 80,000 chemicals have not been adequately tested for their effects on human health." These are scary statistics!

We are constantly exposed to chemicals, toxins, pesticides, and additives every day and all of these take a negative toll on our health. Scientists don't yet know why some people seem to be unaffected when others are impacted so terribly. Perhaps it is because we all have a different "tipping point" in our lives when our body, mind, and emotions just can't take anymore. Perhaps it is how much we are exposed to. Or maybe it is dependent upon our diet or genetics. It doesn't really matter why; the fact is that each of us carry a toxic load that needs to be dealt with.

In an article in *Trends in Endocrinology and Metabolism* (Aug 1, 2017, Vol 28, Issue 8, p. 541-636) it is stated that the "escalating rate of diabetes correlates with global industrialization and the production of plastics, pesticides, synthetic fertilizers, electronic waste, and food additives that release endocrine-disrupting chemicals (EDCs) into the environment and the food chain. Emerging evidence indicates an association between exposure of EDCs and diabetes. In humans, these chemicals are also metabolized by the gut microbiota and thereby their toxicodynamic are altered."

Study after study has examined the effect of pesticides, herbicides, and persistent organic pollutants both individually and as a whole and they have found that the higher the level, the more likely the person was to develop type 2 diabetes, as they cause metabolic and mitochondrial dysfunction. According to an article in *Diabetologia* "these endocrine disrupting chemicals have been shown to do everything from slash insulin levels and raise serum glucose to set-off hyperinsulinemia, worsen glucose tolerance, and insulin sensitivity and reduce insulin-stimulated glucose uptake. The chemicals are also capable of altering the expression of genes, which in at least one study led to a rise in blood glucose levels analogous to those seen in adult-onset diabetes."

We know these products impact our gut microbiota, our cell's ability to function properly, and our hormones, but what can we do to reduce the effects?

While we can't avoid all chemicals, pesticides, toxins, and pollutants, there are a few things that we can do to mitigate our risk:

- ❖ Drink water to assist your body in removing these substances.
- ❖ Eat fibrous vegetables to aid the body in elimination.
- ❖ Use organic nontoxic laundry soap, cleaners, and dish soap.
- ❖ Use an air filter to clean the air in your home, especially in the bedrooms.
- ❖ Avoid using air fresheners or artificial scents.
- ❖ Add a good probiotic to your daily supplement regimen.
- ❖ Avoid using pesticides in your home and yard and if you must use them, use organic nontoxic products.

Managing type 2 diabetes requires more than just changing our diet, we need to change the way we live our lives to ensure we are the healthiest possible.

Medication

Your doctor may prescribe medication to lower your glucose levels, increase sensitivity to insulin, increase production of insulin, or to allow you to lose weight.

Common medications are metformin, sulfonylureas, glinides, thiazolidinediones, DDP-4 inhibitors, GLP-1 receptor agonists, SGLT2 inhibitors, and insulin therapy. Please understand that drug manufacturers have many names for these medications, and the names will change over time. Below is a brief description of the most common types.

Some women find that using medication in addition to a change in diet and lifestyle is very effective and they can be weaned off the medication over time. Other women find the side effects too disruptive and choose to only use a natural approach. You will need to discuss your situation with your doctor to determine what is best for you.

Metformin seems to be the first medication most doctors turn to. It works by lowering the glucose produced in the liver and by improving the body's sensitivity to insulin. Side effects may include: B12 and Co Q10 deficiency, nausea, abdominal pain, bloating, and diarrhea. Some women get all the side effects while others have one or two. Many find the side effects fade over time.

Sulfonylureas helps your body to produce more insulin. Possible side effects include weight gain and low blood sugar.

Glinides help your pancreas to secrete more insulin. They tend to be faster acting than sulfonylureas. Side effects may be weight gain and low blood sugar.

Thiazolidinediones make the body tissue more sensitive to insulin. Side effects may include risk of congestive heart failure, risk of bladder cancer, risk of bone fractures, high cholesterol, and weight gain.

DDP-4 Inhibitors help reduce blood sugar levels, but I have heard it is only slightly effective. Side effects include a risk of pancreatitis and joint pain.

GLP-1 receptor agonists are injectable medications that slow digestion and help to reduce blood sugar levels. They are often used for weight loss and may reduce the risk of heart attack and stroke. Side effects include risk of pancreatitis, nausea, vomiting, and diarrhea.

SGLT2 Inhibitors affect the functioning of the kidneys by slowing return of glucose to the bloodstream, therefore glucose is excreted in the urine. Possible side effects include risk of amputation, risk of bone fractures, risk of gangrene, yeast infections, urinary tract infections, low blood pressure, and high cholesterol.

Insulin therapy used to be a last resort, but many doctors are prescribing this sooner if diet and lifestyle changes do not produce the desired results. There are different types of insulin (long acting, short acting, injectable) and your doctor will determine what is appropriate for you. Side effects of insulin therapy include risk of low blood sugar (hypoglycemia), diabetic ketoacidosis and high triglycerides. Some find it difficult to gauge the exact amount of insulin needed each time, creating anxiety and frustration. There is also a movement of doctors, nutritionists, and scientists that believe just forcing the glucose from the blood stream into the cells isn't enough as it doesn't reduce the overall amount of insulin in the body, just moves it around.

Supplements

A word of caution before taking any supplements—supplements are not regulated the way medicine is and can have potentially dangerous interactions with specific medications. Advertisements for supplements do not have to follow the same rules and regulations that medication does, so just because the advertisement says it does something, does not mean it will give you the results you think it will. Although most supplements are natural products, they are still medicinal in nature, and you can get sick from taking them. Do not take a supplement without first speaking to your doctor or pharmacist.

There are many different supplements you might hear about to aid in regulating your blood sugar, help cells respond better to insulin, or to assist in weight loss. Here are a few of the more common ones:

American Ginseng: May improve our cells response to and body's production of insulin. You need to take it about two hours before each main meal. American Ginseng should never be taken by someone on blood thinners as it can interfere with this type of medication. It may also boost the immune system, so if you are on immunosuppressant drugs, do not take American Ginseng.

Aloe Vera: Supplements made from the plant or juice may help lower fasting blood sugar levels by stimulating insulin production in the pancreas. Studies have not conclusively shown that aloe vera works in this manner. It can interfere with several medications, especially heart medication.

Alpha-Lipoic Acid (ALA): Is actually an antioxidant produced by our liver and is found in some foods such as spinach, red meat, and broccoli. It may improve insulin sensitivity and oxidative damage caused by high blood sugar, although studies show it may take months to experience these effects. ALA interferes with medications for hyperthyroid and hypothyroidism.

Berberine: Studies have shown taking berberine (along with a healthy diet and exercise) reduced fasting blood sugar levels and may help diabetes medication to work better. They believe it helps to improve insulin sensitivity, but it may also cause gas, digestive issues, diarrhea, or constipation. Some find this supplement easier to handle than Metformin.

Chromium: A chromium deficiency reduces our ability to use carbohydrates for energy, which increases our need for more insulin. It may support the cells of the pancreas that create insulin. Antacids, heartburn medications, and other medicine may reduce the absorption of chromium. It is a trace mineral, so it is not needed in large amounts and is available in a variety of foods.

Cinnamon: Yes, the stuff we bake with! Studies show it may help to lower blood sugar and control diabetes. They believe cinnamon helps our cells to respond better to insulin. Cinnamon comes in different types, and the common cassia variety can negatively impact our liver in high doses. Use cinnamon on your oatmeal or a bit in a smoothie but avoid high doses.

Coenzyme Q10: 80 mg daily. It is an antioxidant that improves circulation and stabilizes blood sugar. It works to protect the cells and remove toxins from the body.

Garlic: Decreases and stabilizes blood sugar levels. Enhances immunity and improves circulation. Take a garlic supplement or add fresh garlic to cooking

L-Carnitine: It is thought to mobilize fat. Take 500 mg twice daily on an empty stomach with water (not milk). Take with 50 mg Vitamin B6 or 100 mg Vitamin C for better absorption. L-carnitine plus L-glutamine can reduce sugar cravings.

Probiotics: I always recommend a good probiotic to my clients. Our gut health has a huge impact on our overall health, and poor diet can negatively impact our gut bacteria. Studies have shown probiotics reduce inflammation, improve absorption of nutrition, and may protect the pancreatic cells that make insulin. Probiotics are best taken on an empty stomach, so take it before breakfast or bed.

Manganese: 5 mg daily. Take separately from calcium. This is needed for repair of the pancreas and deficiencies are common in people with diabetes.

Magnesium: 750 mg daily from all supplements. This mineral is used in insulin secretion and absorption by our cells and helps reduce fasting blood sugar levels. Magnesium can interfere with medications such as diuretics, antibiotics, and may cause diarrhea. Always take magnesium with food and avoid magnesium oxide, which can increase the risk of diarrhea.

Vitamin B Complex: 50 mg of each major B Vitamin up to three times daily (do not exceed 300 mg daily) plus extra 50 mg daily of biotin can help improve the metabolism of glucose.

Vitamin D: 400 IU. This fat-soluble vitamin is commonly deficient in the diets of North Americans. It may improve the function of the pancreatic cells that produce insulin and the body's response to it. There are different types of Vitamin D, and your doctor will be able to tell you which type you need and the dose you require. Food sources include cod liver oil, salmon, swordfish, tuna, sardines, beef liver, and it is also now added to fortified orange juice and dairy products because of the deficiency in the general public. Vitamin D is fat soluble and therefore stays in your body longer. Never add a supplement without getting your levels tested first.

Inositol: May help insulin work better, lowers triglycerides, lowers blood pressure, and is often used for people with metabolic disorder and PCOS. There are a lot of people who believe that it may help with depression, panic disorder, bipolar, and PTSD, however, studies do not support this. It may cause gas, diarrhea, and nausea.

Resveratrol: A promising supplement that has shown to improve insulin sensitivity, cardiovascular health, prevent or impede the development of diabetic retinopathy (blindness), and help protect the mitochondria of our cells. High doses of resveratrol may cause stomach upset.

Milk Thistle: Silymarin is an extract from milk thistle and is commonly used to help lower glucose levels, and as a tonic to cleanse the liver. May lead to nausea, vomiting, and diarrhea.

Fenugreek: A seed that may help lower blood glucose levels because it contains fibre and chemicals that help slow down the digestion of carbohydrates and sugars. There is some evidence that it may delay or prevent the onset of type 2 diabetes. Fenugreek can be used as an herb in cooking or be taken as a capsule.

GABA: An amino acid that can help with comfort eating and sugar and carbohydrate cravings caused by stress and anxiety. GABA can help reduce or eliminate stress, anxiety (the stiff muscle and tension type), panic attacks, insomnia (referring to the physical inability to sleep, not the constant thoughts running through your head that keep you awake), and that feeling of having no willpower. Side effects may include sleepiness, upset stomach, headache, and it may decrease blood pressure and cause muscle weakness. GABA may interact with blood pressure medications and anticonvulsants.

Spirulina: A type of blue-green algae with strong antioxidant effects. May help stabilize blood sugar levels. Do not take if you use blood thinners or have an autoimmune condition.

Tryptophan: Helps with sugar cravings, irritability, anxiety, depression (eating to feel happy), and promotes better mood and sleep. L-tryptophan may supress blood glucose levels. Side effects of L-tryptophan may include dizziness, blurred vision, fatigue, hives, nausea, and heart palpitations. Tryptophan can interfere with sedatives, MAO inhibitors, and approximately seventy-five other medications.

Tyrosine: Helps the body build proteins and produce enzymes, thyroid hormones, and helps produce neurotransmitters that aid cells in communication. Found naturally in cheese, beef, lamb, pork, fish, chicken, nuts, eggs, beans, and whole grains which the body converts to dopamine in the gut. May help inhibit insulin secretion from the pancreas. Tyrosine can raise blood pressure rapidly which can lead to a heart attack or stroke and may interfere with thyroid medication.

Zinc: 50 to 80 mg daily (do not exceed 100 mg daily across all supplements). Deficiency has been associated with diabetes. Use zinc gluconate lozenges or OptiZinc for best absorption.

As you can see, there are many herbs, spices, and amino acids that can assist in lowering blood glucose levels, protecting the pancreatic cells, enhancing insulin sensitivity, and helping with cravings. If you make a trip to the local health food store or look online, you will see hundreds of different concoctions that promise to reverse insulin resistance, stop type 2 diabetes, and save us from becoming insulin dependent. As I mentioned earlier, supplements are not regulated the same way medication is, nor are they required to provide proof that their supplement works the way they say it does. In my opinion, I think it's best to add the herbs and spices to your diet to enhance the flavour of your food and obtain the benefits and avoid the pills and powders unless you are working with a nutritionist, dietician, or doctor. Amino acids can be very beneficial but need to be monitored carefully as they can interact with many different medications, so please work with your doctor or pharmacist before adding any to your diet.

Glucose Monitoring

Your doctor may ask you to monitor your blood glucose levels using a glucose monitoring device. These devices can be purchased in most drug stores, department stores (Walmart, Walgreens etc.), as well as online. The type you buy will depend on whether you choose blood or blood-free, the portability of the unit you want, cost, and whether you need a product that is compatible with an insulin pump.

There are many different types of monitors. Blood-free units are usually attached to the upper arm and read bodily fluid instead of blood. They are not considered as accurate as blood-type units but are great for people who hate pricking their fingers. Most glucose monitors include a lancet (for pricking your finger), strips (blood collection), and the unit which measures the glucose in the strip. Some units are higher tech and are implanted under the skin. These will send an alarm if your blood glucose levels fall out of range. New glucose monitoring units are introduced to the market all the time. To determine the type that is best for you, I recommend you speak to your doctor or pharmacist.

Testing can help to determine which foods or activities impact your blood glucose levels. If you are taking insulin, you will need to test your glucose levels before you eat to determine the amount of insulin required. For those who are newly-diagnosed with type 2 diabetes, your doctor may want you to track your glucose levels daily or weekly to determine the success or failure of your ability to lower blood glucose levels as well as which foods send your glucose soaring. Accurate glucose monitoring can be impacted by dehydration, iron anemia, skin products (such as alcohol wipes or antibacterial gel), extreme environmental conditions (such as cold or heat), and, of course, outdated testing strips.

The frequency of testing will be determined by your doctor and will be based on the type of diabetes that you have, what medications you are on, and how many meals you eat per day. In general, testing occurs before each meal, before a workout, and before bed. If you test after a meal you will need to wait one to two hours before testing. Glucose levels are impacted by diet, physical activity, certain medications, illness, injury, dehydration, stress, menopause, menstruation, fatigue, and poor digestion.

While your doctor is the best source of information, for additional information and advice, you can go to the Diabetes Canada or the American Diabetes Association, for information on testing, food recommendations, recipes, and support.

Symptoms of hyperglycemia (high blood sugar) include fatigue, a constant need to urinate, extreme thirst, constantly feeling hungry, loss of weight, and problems with eyesight. Episodes that strike quickly may be caused by a missed meal, too much exercise, or a reaction to too much insulin.

Symptoms of hypoglycemia (low blood sugar) are hunger, dizziness, sweating, confusion, palpitations, and numbness or tingling of the lips. If not treated, the person may experience double vision, trembling, disorientation, and eventually lapse into a coma.

How to Travel Healthy

Eating healthy while travelling can be a challenge for the best of us. I am a nutritionist, and even I have a hard time finding healthy foods in some areas. Preplanning is your lifesaver!

I can recall on a drive from Vancouver, Canada to Ajijic, Mexico, that the highway in Mexico did not have restaurants, and the food available in the gas stations was in my opinion, inedible. I recall going into one gas station which advertised "breakfast now available" in a big sign out front. I was excited until I realized breakfast was a frozen processed egg burrito that was deep fried with a side of tater tots. Other options included row upon row of packages of cookies, muffins, pastries, chips, or candy. Sigh! As a person with type 2 diabetes, you need to plan your meals more thoroughly than the average person.

Car trip

When you are on a road trip, bring a cooler, ice pack, refillable water bottles, and coffee mugs (to avoid drinking out of Styrofoam, which has been linked to cancer and other illness). Go to the grocery stores before you leave, and each night or morning before you start driving. That being said be aware some jurisdictions do not allow you to carry certain foods across their borders. USA and Mexico both ask about fruit, therefore you may need to purchase this once you cross the border.

Bring handy wipes and perhaps a blanket for a picnic as it is always nice to get out and stretch your legs. Also, bring a garbage bag for your waste and dispose of it properly. On a side note, please do not feed scraps to animals as it may have negative implications. For example, wild mountain goats cannot eat lettuce (it is toxic to them) and bears can become brazen if they learn to eat human food. Even wild birds cannot digest breadcrumbs due to the preservatives and chemicals contained in it.

Start your day with a healthy breakfast that will keep you full for several hours. If you consume coffee and a muffin at the hotel, you will be starving in a couple of hours, your blood sugar will be high from the processed food (which is always high in sugar), and you will be searching for food where there may not be any healthy options.

You can always carry unsweetened plain instant oatmeal and small containers of ground flaxseed with cinnamon for a quick filling breakfast for those days when healthy options are not available. Every breakfast bar at a hotel will provide hot water so you can make your instant oatmeal. Most hotels have a few breakfast items such as eggs, fruit, or oatmeal that can be a healthy option. Avoid the processed breads (Danish, bagels, muffins), processed sausages, waffles, or cereal as these foods are loaded with sugar and poor-quality ingredients.

Some foods you can easily carry with you in the car are nuts/seeds, cheese, fruit, and raw cut-up vegetables. Pack your own sandwiches using healthier bread, vegetables, and meat. Plan healthy rest stops along the way by researching restaurants and menus. Almost everything is available online now and it only takes a few minutes of planning to make eating healthy easier. Be wary of packing anything that must be kept very cold as your ice pack will melt eventually.

Subway is a pretty good option, and you can usually find them fairly close to the highway. They have soups, salads, protein bowls, and sandwiches and allow you to add loads of vegetables. If you choose to have a sandwich, tell them to scoop some of the bread out and add a bit of creamy avocado for a healthy fat. Add more vegetables, but stay away from red meats (bacon, salami, pepperoni, ham). A little hint, if you ask for lettuce first, you will get a lot of lettuce, and very few other vegetables—ask for the other vegetables first, and then tell them to add lettuce.

While travelling in the United States, I found Love's Truck Stop carries hard boiled eggs, raw vegetables, fruit, protein cups, and some other healthy options. Super handy if you are stopping for gas and want to get some quick food for the road. Every Love's I stopped at also had a subway attached, which made it very convenient.

McDonald's no longer offers healthy options such as oatmeal or salads, which is very sad for me because I like their coffee. After the documentary "Super Size Me" they did add healthier options, but in the last year or so they have since removed them. Wendy's restaurants still offer salads, but be cautious of the taco chips, dried fruit, and crouton toppings they include with the salads. You can ask for your salad without the toppings, or just scoop them off yourself.

When you stop for the night, make an effort to find a restaurant that serves healthy options (after all, you have been travelling all day and deserve a nice meal). Stock up on more fruits and vegetables for the next day at a grocery store and do not forget to put your ice pack in the freezer and collect it the morning. I have forgotten more ice packs than I can count!

Air travel

I always travel with food on a plane; partly because I do not like the items they serve in those tiny trays, but mostly because I like to be prepared. While on a return flight from the Dominican Republic, the airport had delay after delay after delay. There were so many flights delayed at the airport that all the restaurants had run out of food. When we were finally up in the air, the flight attendant announced they would be serving food, so after confirming the food was coming right out, the gentlemen next to my daughter went to the washroom to give himself his injection of insulin (he was insulin dependent diabetic).

Normally injections are given fifteen to thirty minutes before a meal. Thirty minutes came and went, and the man asked the flight attendant again when the food was coming out. Again, she advised in just a few minutes. Another fifteen minutes went by, and the poor man was starting to sweat. Again, he spoke to her and advised her that he is diabetic and had taken his insulin and that he needed to eat now. She smiled, walked away, and did nothing. Another fifteen minutes went by, and this poor fellow was sweating and shaking and looked like he was about to pass out. My young daughter, who was sitting next to him, timidly asked him if he was okay. Then she told me what was going on. Mom to the rescue! I pulled out cut up oranges, nuts, a sandwich, and handed them to him. We were not served any food for another hour after this, and by the time they got to our seats, they had run out of food. Always be prepared.

Nuts and seeds, cheese, raw cut up vegetables, and fruit are good choices for the plane. Instant plain oatmeal with no sugar makes a handy breakfast. Just ask for a cup of hot water and an extra cup and spoon. Dump the oatmeal into the cup (you may only need to use half depending on the size of the cup), then add the hot water, stir, and let sit for a minute or so. I will often bring a tiny container of ground flaxseed mixed with cinnamon that I can add on top. Pack your own sandwich or purchase a healthier option at subway and carry it on board. Avoid anything with processed meats or food that must be refrigerated, such as eggs (not to mention they are stinky, and your neighbors will not be happy with you).

Bring your own tea bags so you are not tempted with the soda or alcohol. Drink plenty of water to stay hydrated as air travel can be dehydrating, which can affect your blood sugar levels. Staying hydrated can also help prevent the notorious jetlag.

Cruise line or all-inclusive hotel

All day temptation! Huge buffets of nonstop food full of sugar, salt, and bad fats. But if you know what to look for, you can navigate this. After all, you are there for the fun, not the food.

Bring your own refillable cup with a lid so you always have plenty of water with you, making the nonstop soda and alcohol less tempting. Having your own mug also keeps you from having to drink out of Styrofoam cups and avoids anyone putting anything in your drink. The Environmental Protection Agency recognizes Styrofoam can cause headaches, fatigue, dizziness, confusion, and difficulty concentrating. The World Health Organization considers it a possible human carcinogen. It appears to mimic estrogen in the body, disrupts normal hormone production, and may contribute to thyroid problems.

Tell the staff that you are diabetic and cannot eat salt or fatty foods due to hypertension (I know it might be a lie, but this will allow you to ask for food that is prepared especially for you). Do not be afraid to ask the staff for food that is not covered in sauce, cheese, salt, etc. You are their guest, you paid for this food, and they want you to be happy.

Fill up on the salad bar first, then wait ten minutes before you go back for your main course. Make half your plate vegetables, ¼ a lean protein, and the other ¼ one type of starch. Use smaller plates so you can't over-fill.

If you feel as though you can't have a specific food, it can trigger serious cravings or feelings of being left out. If this is the case, pick one day you will allow yourself to have a dessert or unhealthy food of your choice (providing that your blood sugar levels allow this). Just remember the rules and choose something in the correct portion size of the finest quality and sit and enjoy every bite.

Skip the booze! Seriously, the average woman gains five pounds or more in one week at an all-inclusive hotel between the free drinks and never-ending food. Alcohol not only causes your blood sugar to rise, but can also mask low blood sugar, making it dangerous for those with hypoglycemia. Alcohol can stimulate your appetite and impair your willpower, making junk food more appealing. Excessive alcohol can also increase your chances of tripping and getting injured or of making you sleep the next day away with a hangover.

I met a young woman who got drunk in Playa Del Carmen and fell down a flight of stairs. She spent the first night of her dream vacation in the emergency room at the local hospital and the next five days with her foot up in the shade or hobbling around on crutches while her friends went parasailing, snorkelling, explored ancient ruins, and toured the jungle in a dune buggy. Skip the alcohol, stay safe, get up the next morning, and spend the day having fun and making memories.

If you do choose to drink alcohol, make sure your blood sugar levels are stable first. Only drink alcohol with food, avoid sugary mixed drinks (those mixed with fruit juice or heavy cream), drink slowly, and try to limit yourself to only one drink per day. If you choose to have more than one drink, try drinking a bottle of water in between.

Shift Work

Recent statistics indicate the majority of the working population is engaged in irregular or "non-standard" working hours, including shifts and nights, weekends, split shifts, on-call, compressed weeks, telework, part-time, variable/flexible working time, and prolonged duty periods (12+ hour shifts.)

Working nights is a particular problem as humans were designed to sleep at night when it is dark, and wake during daylight hours. Working nights interferes with the natural biological functions that are activated during the day and supressed at night. Shiftwork places stress on workers who are constantly adjusting to a new sleep schedule and to their family members who are on a regular daytime schedule.

The misalignment of circadian rhythms of body functions is responsible for the so-called "jetlag" (or "shift-lag," in this case) syndrome, characterized by feelings of fatigue, sleepiness, insomnia, digestive troubles, irritability, poorer mental agility, and reduced performance. Women who sleep less than six hours have a higher chance of insulin resistance and obesity.

After a night shift, workers usually go to bed as soon as they get home, that is one or two hours after the end of the shift, depending on commuting time and family commitments (which are typically greater for women). This means they have to sleep during the biological rising phase which sustains wakefulness—this makes it difficult to fall and stay asleep. Also, because the environmental conditions are not the most appropriate, noises and bright light can cause sleep to be further disturbed. Consequently, sleep is often reduced by several hours, it is interrupted more frequently, and the much-needed stage two and REM (rapid eye movement) sleep is commonly not achieved. This makes the worker feel more tired.

The second most common complaint for shift workers (after fatigue) is digestive issues. This is due to the timing disruption between mealtimes and the normal circadian phases of our gastrointestinal functions (for example gastric, bile, and pancreatic secretions, enzyme activity, rate of absorption of nutrients, leptin, and ghrelin hormones), as well as the difference in the foods eaten during shift work, which tend to be more processed and higher in sugar and salt content. We also generally drink soda. Basically, because our body was designed to be active when the sun comes up, more active in the afternoon, and start to slow down as the sun sets, followed by a period of feeling sleepy and getting ready to sleep—shift work interferes with the natural functions of the body.

The most common complaints are constipation, indigestion, gas, irritable bowel syndrome, and metabolic syndromes (obesity, high cholesterol, insulin imbalance).

Shift workers are more likely to eat processed high sugar foods and drinks to stay awake, especially on long shifts or when there has been an inadequate break between shift schedule changes. Soda, chocolate bars, chips, and candy are popular vending machine items in areas shift workers are located, feeding the need for a boost in energy. High sugar diets not only spike our insulin but also feed the bad bacteria in our gut, causing inflammation and illness to flourish as well as causing the sugar highs and crashes that prompt the need for further stimulants.

In 1999, Knutsson and Boggild reviewed seventeen studies and concluded there is evidence of a strong association between shift workers having on average 40% excess risk for ischemic heart disease as compared to day workers. This is due to the correlation between the stress related to the sleep cycle and circadian disruption, sleep deprivation, work and family conflicts, and lack of healthy eating and exercise.

So, what's a girl to do? You probably can't quit your job to avoid shift work but there are a few things that you can do to ensure better health. The most important one is to change what you are eating. Avoid processed food, soda, and other junk that is commonly eaten to provide an instant energy boost. These foods may give you a quick boost but the sugar crash that follows will just have you reaching for more. Instead, take your meals and eat fruit, berries, and vegetables for energy and nourishment. Eat fibrous foods such as raw vegetables, salads, and high-quality grains that will keep you feeling full longer and promote continuous energy over a long period of time. Eat healthy lean protein such as eggs, grass fed hormone-free poultry, nuts, and seeds, as well as fish to help you stay full and provide much-needed amino acids. Take a water bottle so you have clean water to sip on throughout your shift. Take digestive enzymes with meals for the first month or so until the heart burn, gas, and indigestion have passed. Each day, before you sleep, take a probiotic on an empty stomach.

This will require not only planning out your meals, snacks, and drinks for your work period, but also for the rest of your day. When we are fatigued, we are more likely to reach for highly-processed instant foods to "fill the stomach or give us energy" rather than expending energy to think of healthier options. This is especially true if you are cooking for your family while sleep deprived. Ask other family members to pitch in to help with meal preparation, cooking healthy meals and shopping for healthy foods. Remember, you don't have to be Superwoman.

The second thing you must focus on is getting sufficient sleep. Wear an eye mask and use black out curtains to simulate nighttime. Wear ear plugs and/or use white noise to block out daytime noise. Turn off your phone so you are not interrupted by ringing or message indicator lights. You may find that a warm bath or meditation before you go to bed can help you fall asleep faster.

Ask family and friends to pitch in to help with childcare or other activities so that you can get the required amount of sleep. Avoid nicotine, alcohol, exercise, and watching television before going to bed as these may interfere with a good sleep. Get a good-quality mattress and pillow and keep the bedroom cool. If your partner works a different shift and you wake each other up due to your different schedules, you may find separate bedrooms helpful so you can each get a good night's sleep.

Sleep aids, such as supplemental melatonin or other medications, can interfere with our natural rhythm. While it is helpful on a short-term, temporary basis, if you are travelling or suffering from temporary insomnia, it is not something I recommend as a long-term solution. Instead, try increasing foods that contain the amino acid "tryptophan," such as poultry, eggs, dairy, nuts, and seeds. Tryptophan becomes serotonin in the body, which then becomes melatonin. By increasing our natural intake of tryptophan, we can help our body create the necessary melatonin for proper sleep.

Sleep is essential to our health and is not something we can skip or shortchange ourselves on. We need it to be healthy physically, mentally, and emotionally, not just for ourselves, but for our family as well. The average person needs eight hours of sleep per day however children may need ten, and those who have an illness may need up to twelve hours a day. Ironically, we often reduce our sleep time in favor of other activities so we can "get more done," which can cause increased chance of illness in the long-run. And while we are on the subject, it is almost impossible to "catch up" on sleep on your day off and to "bank sleep" for later. Our body just doesn't work that way. Each period of sleep gives the opportunity for healing, digestion, and cell repair, and research has shown that an hour of missing sleep can take up to four days to recover from. If you are sleep deprived all week, you will not be able to catch up on your sleep on one day off. Get the proper sleep each night and make it a priority to do so as part of your healthy lifestyle.

Children

When your child is first diagnosed with type 2 diabetes, it is a terrifying feeling, and as parents we want to do everything in our power to help our child. Visions of limb amputations, blindness, and stroke flash through our minds. We blame ourselves and vow to do anything we can to change this, but if there is one thing I have learned, it is that blame does not help. The only thing that helps is knowledge, a plan, and the dedication to make the necessary changes to ensure the health of your child.

The rise of type 2 diabetes in children is staggering. In the mid 1990s (at the same time as genetically-engineered food full of high fructose corn syrup reached the market), the rate of childhood obesity and type 2 diabetes began to rise each year. According to an article in the World Journal of Diabetes, most children with type 2 diabetes are obese or extremely obese at diagnosis. Obesity has an adverse effect on glucose metabolism, and obese children have higher amounts of insulin in their blood than normal children—they also have approximately 40% lower insulin-stimulated glucose metabolism (the ability of the cells to use insulin) compared with non-obese children. In addition, the more visceral fat (the fat around the organs), the more insulin sensitivity in the child.

Risk factors for developing diabetes include family history, excess weight, sedentary lifestyle, high blood pressure, high cholesterol, and low-income status (due to inadequate access to fresh fruits, vegetables, and lean proteins). Children of families of lower economic status have less access to healthy meals, and are more dependent on processed cheaper foods, which as I explained earlier in this book, are lower in nutrition and higher in sugar, salt, and chemicals. These children additionally have less access to safe play areas, recreational centers, and have higher rates of television and screen time.

Culture affects our body weight and perceptions of what is normal. From the time we are little we look to our parents and extended family to learn what is normal. In some cultures, gaining weight is healthy, and children of normal weight are "too skinny." Being overweight may be associated with strength, wealth, and fertility and if other members of the family are overweight or obese, the child is more likely to gain weight to fit into the family dynamic. There may also be a well-meaning friend or relative that is always pushing food or encouraging your child to eat more. Maybe a grandparent or auntie who will not let them leave their house without eating something?

Food pushers are a real thing and dealing with them can be a bit tricky. On the one hand, you don't want to upset your well-meaning family member, but on the other hand you have the health and well-being of your child to consider. Here are a few tips that might help you. Option A is to not visit during mealtimes (this usually gets you out of several helpings of a meal). Tell them you just ate (be warned, they will tell you it isn't as good as theirs so you need more and want to give you food), and if they push food on you, tell them you would love to take it home to eat it later. Then ask for a glass of water so you have something in your hand. Option B is to explain that your doctor has advised your child needs to follow a specific diet. Truthfully, this one is a bit harder because they will argue that their food is healthy, and they know better than the doctor. Option C is to explain low glycemic eating and how this affects blood sugar levels, so the family is now only eating certain foods. Honestly, trying to convince someone else that their eating habits are unhealthy is very difficult without insulting them. For children this can be impossible, and they end up feeling pressured to conform.

Depending on your child's medical situation, your doctors may prescribe metformin or similar drugs to help reduce weight, while other doctors realize the long-term negative effect of these medications and choose to instead work with the family to create a healthier lifestyle to naturally manage this syndrome. If you are uncomfortable with your doctor's recommendations, you are entitled to a second opinion. Always work with your doctor and never restrict the calories of a child without consulting their doctor first. Children are still growing and have certain caloric needs depending on their age and growth cycle. It is quite common for physicians to keep them at their current caloric intake and allow them to "grow into" the caloric range rather than limiting calories.

It is not enough to change the diet and lifestyle of one child in your home—remember, this is a lifestyle change for the whole family. We don't want to single out one member, making them feel responsible for the other members of the family. If you don't allow ice cream into the house because one child is prediabetic, the other child may make comments about the lack of ice cream, making the sick child feel responsible or unhappy and the healthy child resentful of the sick one. While the majority of the time, the food in the household needs to be healthy, allow the occasional treat to accommodate all members of the home. If your child is insulin dependent, the "treat" may need to be discussed with their doctor in order to keep their blood sugar balanced. But remember to make this a rare occasion. Most of the diet needs to be based on healthy, low glycemic foods without added sugars or anything processed. As a parent, you need to set the example for your child. If the parent is eating and drinking unhealthy food on a regular basis, then so will the child. If the parent is eating healthy and exercising, then the child is more likely to follow suit. Remember, they want to be like you, and as the adult you must lead by example.

It is important to talk about the language you use for yourself. If you are constantly talking about your latest diet, or that you are fat or hate your body, then the child will adopt the same attitude. We have far more influence on our young children than we realize. When you are talking about your own eating habits, use the same words that you would for your child. Talk about exercising for strength and agility, about eating for stronger bones or muscles. Use words of love and acceptance to describe your body rather than talking about having to lose ten pounds so you look good in a bathing suit or to fit into a specific size of clothing. Language matters, and they are listening.

Portion size and number of portions are dependent on the age of the child, their size, and growing periods. Sometimes they are fussy and don't want to eat a particular food but may accept it at a later time, so don't give up too easily as it takes multiple exposures to a specific food before it is accepted by a child. Children also have more taste buds than adults, so a food may seem too bitter, salty, or spicy for them even if it tastes fine for us, so keep food a bit blander. Serve fresh vegetables, whole grains, lean protein, and fruit and do not serve food that is high in sugars, preservatives, or food additives. Limit deep-fried foods and processed snack foods. Do not use food as a reward or bribe, only as nourishment. Using sweet food as a reward teaches them that sweet food is desirable while healthy food is not. Teach them early that food is for nourishment, not for comfort, reward, or punishment.

Toddlers are very good at knowing when they have had enough to eat, and you should never shove food in their mouth to force them to eat more. They will give you cues such as turning their head away, gagging, crying, spitting out the food, or trying to leave the table. Never force a child to finish what is on their plate. As adults, we often give too much and worry that they aren't eating enough. Aim to give one tablespoon per year for each dish. For example, a three-year-old would receive three tablespoons of food for the meal. Serve healthy snacks in between mealtimes rather than having the child only eat three meals a day. Most young children are grazers by nature and although we may worry they aren't eating enough, they will consume enough food throughout the day. Toddlers should not have more than ½ a cup of fruit juice a day and I recommend watering it down so there is less sweetness to it. Juice should never be left in a bottle in the crib or out for them to sip on over a longer period as this will promote tooth decay. If you choose to give them juice, serve it at the table and remove it when they are done.

For children ages four to five, aim to provide three servings of vegetables (portion size 1/2 cup), one serving of fruit (size of a tennis ball), two servings of grains (portion size is 1/2 cup), two servings of milk or alternatives (3/4 of a cup), and two servings of meat or alternatives (portion size is two eggs or size of a deck of cards) throughout the day. This food should be served as three meals and three snacks (some children do not require an evening snack). You may offer ¼ cup of nuts and seeds (not peanuts due to allergies and mold), but only if there is no risk of choking. Also be sure to always watch for allergies.

Ages five to eight will have four servings of vegetables, one serving of fruit or berries, three servings of grains, two servings of milk or alternatives, two servings of protein, and one serving of nuts and seeds. Portion sizes are the same.

From ages nine to eleven increase vegetables to five servings, one serving of fruit or berries, four servings of grains, two servings of milk or alternatives, two to three servings of protein, and one serving of nuts and seeds. Portion sizes are the same.

After the age of twelve, your child will have their own food preferences and the number of portions will vary depending on their height, body size, activity level, and whether they are in a growth period. Aim to provide two servings of fruit or berries, six servings of vegetables, four servings of grains, one serving of nuts and seeds, two servings of protein, and two servings of milk or alternatives. Teenagers need a lot of water! Avoid serving any sugary drinks, flavored milk, energy drinks, sports drinks, and soda.

Many teenagers eat fast foods and snack foods outside the home, which are high in salt, saturated fats, sugars, and preservatives. Encourage them to eat healthy meals and snacks but understand that at this age their peers may have more influence on their eating habits than you do. Provide them healthy meals at home (where you can control their food intake) and teach them to nourish their body outside of the home. Have healthy snacks such as fruit, berries, nuts, and seeds, or raw vegetables available in order to encourage healthy snacking. If kids don't see a quick and easy snack food, they will reach for the unhealthy foods because it is "easy and filling." I found that if there was fruit on the table, and healthy options within eyesight in the fridge already pre-prepared, then my daughter would eat it. If she had to look for something or heaven forbid cut up a melon or wash a vegetable, then I got the "there's nothing to eat!" and she would reach for a cookie or bread.

Depending on the age of your child, changing their diet can be a bit tricky, so start by doing an assessment of what your child eats and drinks in a day when they are with you, at school, or out with friends. How many sugary drinks are they consuming? What are they eating for snacks? How much processed foods are they consuming? What are their portion sizes? Do they eat after dinner right before bed? You may start by sending them to school with a healthier lunch and reducing portion sizes to the proper size and number of portions for their age group. Take out fruit juice and add in whole fruit. Add in more fresh raw vegetables, whole wheat, or rye bread instead of white bread. Switch French fries for sweet potatoes, brown rice, or quinoa. Reduce the amount of packaged and processed foods (such as cereal, pop tarts, snack boxes, noodle soup, etc.) and replace it with healthier options.

You will never be able to control everything your child eats outside of the home as kids trade food, buy it from corner stores, or refuse to eat what you have sent for them. However, you can provide them the healthiest options and explain to them how eating these foods will make them stronger and healthier.

Next, do an assessment of the child's activity level and how much screen time they have each day. How often are they outside playing? What do they do with their friends? Are they involved in sports? Start by limiting screen time (computer, phone, television, and games) to no more than one hour a day. I want to warn you in advance that they will not be happy about this but stick to your choices. Encourage them to get outside to play and be physically active. This may mean playing with them or teaching them to play a sport.

The key to changing a child's behavior is to do this gradually and make it fun so they don't feel they are being penalized because of their health. Start doing activities that everyone enjoys, such as playing basketball or soccer, going for walks, riding bicycles, swimming, or walking the dog. If your child's friends are also inactive, you can either encourage all of them to be more active or enroll your child in an activity without their current friends.

Children need an hour of exercise per day, whether it is organized sports, walking, playing outside, household chores, or activities with family members. Remember, the more fun you make it the more they will want to participate. Young children are more likely to want to participate if you are involved. They will follow your example, so if you are sitting on the computer or watching television then so will they.

Never yell, bribe, punish, or threaten your child about their weight, food, or exercise. If these issues turn into fights, the results can be harmful. The worse kids feel about their weight the more likely they are to binge eat or develop an eating disorder. Remember, food is nutrition and should never be used as a punishment or reward. Do not send them to bed without dinner if they misbehave or promise a sweet treat for a good report card. It is important to establish that food is only for nutrition, not comfort, reward, or punishment. Compliment them when they choose a healthier option such as playing basketball outside rather than sitting and watching television, but do not focus on weight loss. Let this change be all about being healthier as a family, and not about the weight loss.

Limit sugary drinks and encourage children to drink more water. I have seen many children drinking pop and have even witnessed mothers putting soda in a baby bottle. Children should not be drinking soda as it increases the risk of obesity, dental cavities, fatty liver disease, and kidney disease. A child size Coca-Cola from McDonalds has one-hundred calories and twenty-six grams of sugar. That is over six teaspoons of sugar in one drink. Children should never be drinking energy drinks as the added caffeine can make them extremely ill. Switch them to drinking milk (depending on the age of the child), or water. They may complain about not having their favourite soda or fruit juice in the house, but they will adapt. Get them a really cool water bottle that encourages them to drink more water.

Limit the amount of screen time to no more than one hour for children over two years and under twelve, and two hours (including homework time) for children aged thirteen to eighteen. Television is especially troublesome as it is full of advertisements for processed foods and drinks that will encourage unhealthy behaviors. Studies are showing that increased screen time has negative effects on the brain and social development of young children. Excessive screen time has been linked to aggressive behavior when the device is taken away, an inability to understand nonverbal social cues, eye strain, and, of course, obesity.

Encourage them to eat fresh whole fruits such as apples, bananas, or oranges. Buy fruits in season to lower the cost. Switch from white bread to whole wheat and stop buying boxed cereals. Have them eat eggs or oatmeal for breakfast. Provide them extra vegetables and leafy greens and fewer processed carbohydrates. Serve smaller portion sizes, as they are not adults and do not need the same size or number of servings as an adult.

Encourage children to try new types of fruits and vegetables. It may take several tries before your child likes a certain food, but sometimes changing the way we serve it (raw, steamed, baked, broiled) determines whether they will like it. At a later point, do not be afraid to try a food they previously did not like; for years my daughter hated mushrooms and tomatoes, and now she likes them. Kids!

Improve your child's quality of sleep by ensuring a regular bedtime that allows them to have eight to ten hours of sleep per night. Stop all electronics at least an hour before bedtime, shut off any electronics in their room to stop any blue light (this interferes with sleep), and make the room dark and quiet. If you live in a noisy neighborhood, try playing white sound in the background using a fan. Remove pets from the bedroom (especially those that are active at night), as children are more susceptible to pet dander and allergies.

Making these changes all at once can be overwhelming, so start with two or three at a time. Stop buying fruit juice or soda and buy whole fruit instead. Make them oatmeal with berries or scrambled eggs with spinach instead of giving them a sugary boxed cereal. Serve raw vegetables and dip on movie nights instead of chips. Stop buying pop tarts and cookies and put a fruit bowl on the table.

Depending on the age of the child, you can create a healthier lifestyle plan together. Make sure you listen to their ideas and incorporate some of them into your plan. This will create "buy in" and will make your child want to participate more. Let them choose a new fruit or vegetable to try at the grocery store. Look up healthy recipes together and teach them to cook.

Talk with your child about their weight and encourage them to share their feelings and thoughts. Make sure you are actively listening; if you have had similar experiences, it might help to share them. Reassure them that you love them no matter what size they are, and always will. Use language such as "we are going to get healthier as a family" not "you are on a diet." Describe foods as healthy, or that this food gives us strong bones, or this food gives us good eyesight. Do not describe food as "bad" or "fattening" as this may create an unhealthy relationship with food. Children tend to equate behaviors with self-esteem. For example, because they eat "bad" food they are bad. Or because they eat "fattening" food they are fat. You get the idea. Language is important!

They say it takes a village to raise a child. Making healthy changes in the home can be difficult for low-income families, single parents, or working parents. Why not include other family members? Neighbors? Perhaps you can join together to bring about positive change for everyone?

I know of one family who had difficulty ensuring their child ate healthily or was active after school because they worked until dinner time. The parents felt there was nothing they could do until they spoke to an elderly neighbor who said she would love to have their child in her home after school. She would provide a healthy snack and play with the child and in exchange the parents agreed to walk the neighbor's dog in the evening when it was too dark for her to leave the house. It was a win! Not only did the child get exercise before dinner but the whole family went for a walk with the dog in the evening. Perhaps there is an option for a community garden? I have often found once ideas get flowing, there is no end to the wonderful solutions that can be found.

If your child suffers from hyperglycemia or hypoglycemia or is insulin dependent, you must ensure that your child's teacher and the school is informed. Provide any medication or glucose tablets, hard candy, or fruit juice as appropriate. Make sure the staff know the signs of low blood sugar and to never leave your child alone after treatment. Symptoms include shakiness, hunger, sweating, dizziness, irritability, pale skin, sudden behavioral changes, trouble paying attention, confusion, or confusion upon awakening.

Conclusion

I have witnessed amazing transformations resulting from creating a healthier diet and lifestyle. People who were overweight, depressed, suffered from constant fatigue, and were dependent upon medication, are now slimmer, more energetic, and medication-free. They have gone from worrying about the future to looking forward to a bright and happy tomorrow. While it does take time and effort, it is worth the short-term work for such important gain. You deserve to have a long and healthy life without fear of illness or disease. You deserve to have a fit and energetic body, now and forever. You deserve to have a bright future.

Managing type 2 diabetes is not only possible but is one of the most important things you can do for yourself and your family. As I have explained in this book, by removing endocrine disruptors, added sugar, processed foods, and deep fried and fast foods, we can balance our hormones and blood glucose levels and heal our body naturally, giving us better health, energy, and vitality.

By creating a better relationship with food, going from one of comfort to one of nutrition, we eliminate guilt and the shame associated with the diet mentality. We have all been trapped in this mindset and feeling that we need to "fix" ourselves; changing our perspective on food is key to changing our health. You no longer need to purchase the latest diet pill, powder, or gimmick and can rest easy knowing you are doing what is best for your body now and in the future.

Getting better sleep and learning to reduce our stress and create healthy habits for work, travel, and at home gives our life more joy and purpose. While I have given you many suggestions and ways to implement new habits and reduce stress in your life, you have made the changes necessary to create a more balanced lifestyle. Some of you may have decided to incorporate all the suggestions while others may only have implemented a few. Whatever you decided, it is my hope that you are able to make the changes necessary to create a balanced lifestyle that works for you.

I hope you have enjoyed this book and have discovered ways to naturally manage your type 2 diabetes, giving yourself a brighter, healthier future. Before you go, I need your help. It will only take a few minutes of your precious time. If you enjoyed this book, can you take a few minutes of your valuable time and give a rating on the book from wherever you purchased it (Amazon Kindle, Kobo, Barnes & Noble etc.)?

To thank you for taking the time out of your busy schedule to provide a rating on this book; I would like to gift you *30 Motivational Tips* to help keep you focused on your goals. Log in to www.powerfulevenutrition.com and download for free from the book section.

If you or someone you know needs more help changing their diet and lifestyle, please feel free to contact me at info@powerfulevenutrition.com and we can discuss ways to help you get the life and health that you deserve.

And finally, please follow me on Facebook at www.facebook.com/powerfulevenutrition for more health and lifestyle tips, recipes, and information on a variety of subjects.

List of low-medium glycemic index foods
(Note: this list is not exhaustive but an example)

- Most non-starchy vegetables (exp. asparagus, broccoli, cauliflower, cucumber, lettuce, peppers, mushrooms, celery, kale, onions, spinach, squash, tomatoes)
- Peas, chickpeas, beans (green, kidney, red), lentils
- Pearl barley
- Peaches, kiwi fruit, apple, pear, banana, plum, grapefruit, cherries, oranges
- Whole wheat spaghetti
- Cooked carrots
- Sweet potatoes
- Long grain brown rice
- Couscous
- Oatmeal
- Soy milk
- Eggs
- Chicken breast, cod, turkey breast, shrimp, haddock
- Dijon mustard, apple cider vinegar, red wine vinegar, balsamic vinegar, most spices, garlic

List of foods to avoid

- White potatoes, corn
- White bread
- White rice
- White pasta
- Barbecue sauce, marinara sauce, canned pasta sauces, ketchup, teriyaki,
- Sweet relish, honey mustard,
- Processed meats (salami, bacon, ham, beef jerky, sausage)
- Processed baked goods
- Processed snack goods (microwave popcorn, chips, cookies)
- Sweetened breakfast cereals
- Dried fruits and canned fruit
- Deep fried foods (French fries, onion rings)
- Higher fat cuts of meat (brisket, prime rib, rib-eye steak)
- Anything with trans fats
- Sugary foods (candy, cookies, cake, cotton candy)
- Sweetened drinks (fruit juice, sports drinks, sweetened tea).

Green Smoothie Recipe

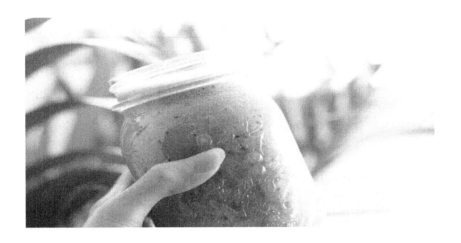

2 cups of water (or unsweetened green tea)
2 cups lettuce (red, romaine or leafy green)
2 cups spinach or kale
1 tbsp ground flaxseed
3 low glycemic fruits (either 1 cup or 1 medium sized fruit – seedless)
1 medium avocado

1. Add water to blender. Chop greens and add to blender. Add flaxseed, avocado, chopped fruit.
2. Blend until liquid. Can add ice if you prefer cold.
3. Drink immediately, or store in fridge up to 2 days or freeze.

Healthy Meal Plan

I know that changing our diet and lifestyle can be challenging to say the least. We have the best of intentions but making huge changes can be overwhelming, causing some of you to give up. I want to make healthy eating an easy lifestyle change.

The following *Healthy Meal Plan* is a six week dietary plan designed to allow you to transition from the Standard American Diet high in carbohydrates and added sugars, to a healthier low glucose eating plan.

Each week the recipes will reduce inflammatory foods and assist in healing digestive health. Options to the recipes may be included to add various spices, vegetarian options, or alternative ingredients. Please be aware that recipes are provided only one time even if they are used on multiple weeks.

By following the *Healthy Meal Plan* your eating habits will be changed allowing you to have the greatest success in whichever diet you choose to follow.

At the end of the six week *Healthy Meal Plan* you will need to decide how you wish to proceed. In the last chapter, I outline both the ketogenic and low glycemic carbohydrate plans proving you with the pros and cons of each style.

Healthy Meal Plan: Week One

Week one: is low sugar, low glycemic and lower calories but higher in healthy fats to keep you feeling fuller. Drink only one cup unsweetened caffeinated coffee/tea. Drink plenty of water, water with lemon, spearmint, and red raspberry leaf tea.

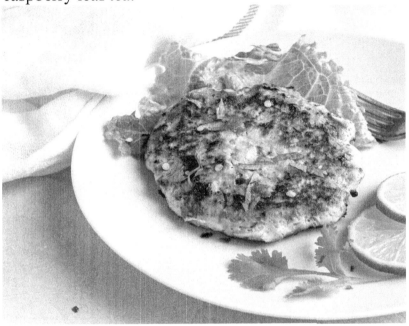

Week One Meal Plan

	Mon	Tue	Wed	Thu	Fri	Sat	Sun
Breakfast	Scrambled Eggs with Peppers & Kale	Blueberries	Spinach & Sweet Potato Egg Muffins	Spinach & Sweet Potato Egg Muffins	Chia Oats with Kiwi	Zucchini Turkey Breakfast Skillet	Greek Yogurt Waffles
		Flax Bread Avocado Toast	Raspberries				Fresh Strawberries
Lunch	Tuna Salad Plate	Turkey & Vegetable Soup	Turkey & Vegetable Soup	Salmon Salad Lettuce Wraps	Ginger Cilantro Salmon Burgers	Greek Chicken Salad	Turmeric Beef Stew
		Whole Wheat Flatbread			Roasted Mini Peppers		
Snack 2	Apple	Hummus Dippers	Bell Peppers with Hummus	Peach & Almonds	Sunbutter Pumpkin Protein Balls	Apple	Celery with Goat Cheese
			Carrot Sticks				
Dinner	Roasted Turkey Breast & Carrots	Steamed White Fish with Tomato & Olive Sauce	Zucchini Noodles with Salmon	Saffron Chicken Kebab with Salad	Saffron Chicken Kebab with Salad	Turmeric Beef Stew	Spaghetti Squash Chow Mein
	House Salad	Steamed Asparagus			Steamed Green Beans		

Scrambled Eggs with Peppers & Kale

5 ingredients · 15 minutes · 1 serving

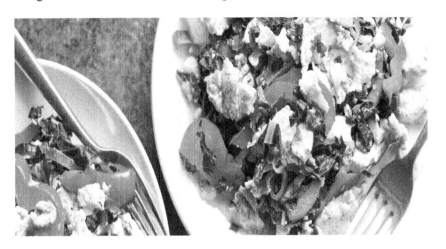

Directions

1. Heat the olive oil in a skillet over medium heat. Add the red bell pepper and kale leaves and sauté until softened, about 5 to 7 minutes.

2. While the veggies are cooking, crack the eggs into a bowl and season with salt and pepper. Beat gently with a fork until well combined.

3. Push the veggies to one side of the pan and pour the beaten eggs into the empty side. Use a spatula to scramble, slowly incorporating the veggies once the eggs are no longer very wet.

Ingredients

3/4 tsp Extra Virgin Olive Oil
1/2 Red Bell Pepper (sliced)
1 cup Kale Leaves (chopped)
3 Egg
Sea Salt & Black Pepper (to taste).

Flax Bread Avocado Toast

4 ingredients · 5 minutes · 1 serving

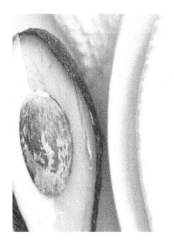 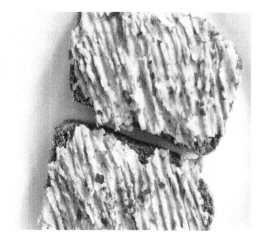

Directions

1. Toast flax bread in toaster, or broil on high for about 3 minutes per side.

2. Mash avocado on bread. Sprinkle red pepper flakes and sea salt. Enjoy!

Ingredients

1 slice Grain-Free Flax Bread

1/4 Avocado

1/16 tsp Red Pepper Flakes

1/16 tsp Sea Salt.

Spinach & Sweet Potato Egg Muffins

8 ingredients · 35 minutes · 2 servings

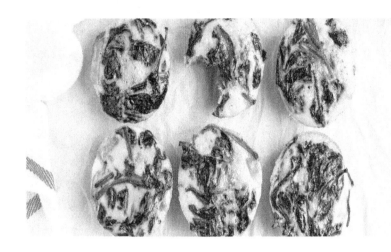

Directions

1. Preheat oven to 350°F (177°C). Lightly grease a muffin pan with avocado oil.

2. Steam sweet potato in a double boiler for 8 to 10 minutes, or until tender when pierced with a fork. Let cool slightly.

3. While the sweet potato is steaming, heat extra virgin olive oil in a large pan over medium heat. Sauté the spinach until wilted and tender. Let cool slightly.

4. When spinach and sweet potatoes are cool enough to handle, divide evenly into the muffin cups of the prepared pan.

5. In a mixing bowl whisk eggs until well scrambled.

Whisk in water and salt and pepper.

6. Pour the whisked eggs into the muffin cups to cover the sweet potato and spinach.

7. Bake for 15 to 18 minutes or just until the egg is cooked through and no longer liquid on top. Remove from oven, let cool and enjoy!

Ingredients

3/4 tsp Avocado Oil
1/2 Sweet Potato (medium, peeled and chopped into cubes)
1 1/2 tsps Extra Virgin Olive Oil
3 cups Baby Spinach
4 Eggs
2 tbsps Water
1/4 tsp Sea Salt
1/4 tsp Black Pepper

Notes

Serving Size
One serving is equal to three egg cups.

Leftovers
Store in the fridge in an airtight container up to three days. Due to the moisture in the sweet potato and spinach, these egg cups do not freeze well.

No Baby Spinach
Use finely sliced kale or Swiss chard instead.

Chia Oats with Kiwi

4 ingredients · 10 minutes · 1 serving

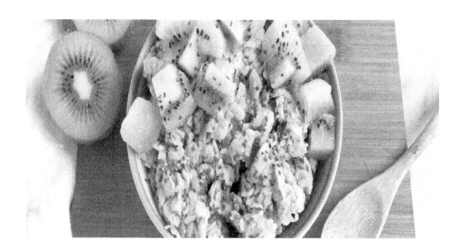

Directions

1. In a small saucepan, bring the water to a boil and add the oats and chia seeds. Reduce to a simmer and cook for 4 to 5 minutes or until cooked through. Be sure to stir often.
2. Divide the oatmeal between bowls and top with kiwi. Enjoy!

Ingredients

1/2 cup Water
1/2 cup Oats (rolled)
1 tbsp Chia Seeds
1/2 Kiwi (chopped)

Notes

Leftovers

Refrigerate in an airtight container for up to four days. For best results, reheat with additional liquid over the stove or in the microwave.

Serving Size

One serving is equal to half a cup of oatmeal and half of a kiwi.

Zucchini Turkey Breakfast Skillet

6 ingredients · 20 minutes · 1 serving

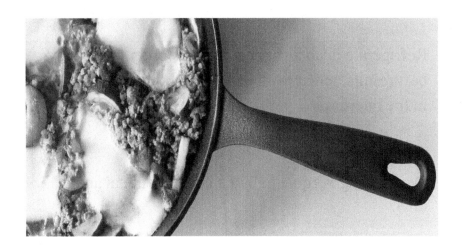

Directions

1. Add the coconut oil to a large skillet and place over medium heat.

2. Cook the ground turkey, breaking it up as it cooks through. Once it starts to brown, stir in the zucchini. Continue to sauté until the zucchini has softened (about 3 - 5 minutes).

3. Add the salsa to the skillet and stir well to mix.

4. Use a spoon to create pockets for the eggs. Crack an egg into each pocket and cover the skillet with a lid. Let the eggs cook until done to your liking (3 to 5 minutes).

5. Divide onto plates and season with sea salt and black pepper to taste. Add hot sauce if you'd like some heat. Enjoy

Ingredients

1/2 tsp Coconut Oil
5 1/3 ozs Extra Lean Ground Turkey
2/3 Zucchini (large, finely diced)
1/3 cup Salsa
1 Egg
Sea Salt & Black Pepper (to taste)

Notes

Vegetarian
Use lentils instead of ground turkey.

More Greens
Stir in baby spinach or kale right after you add the salsa. Stir until wilted.

No Salsa
Use crushed tomatoes instead.

Greek Yogurt Waffles

8 ingredients · 25 minutes · 3 servings

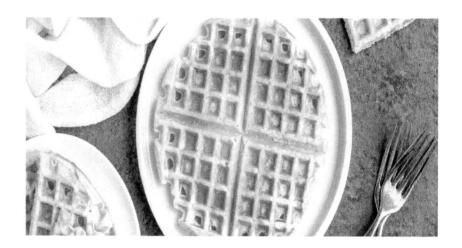

Directions

1. In a mixing bowl, combine the milk, Greek yogurt, egg, and vanilla extract. Whisk in the flour, baking powder, and salt and continue to stir until just combined.

2. Preheat the waffle maker to medium-high heat. Lightly brush the waffle maker with some of the oil. Spoon the batter onto the bottom side of the waffle maker in 1/2 cup portions. Cook the waffles for two to three minutes or until golden brown. Repeat with the remaining batter brushing the waffle maker with more oil between each waffle.

Ingredients

¾ **cup** Cow's Milk, Reduced Fat
5 1/4 tbsps Plain Greek Yogurt
1 Egg
3/4 tsp Vanilla Extract
1 cup Unbleached All Purpose Flour
2 tsp Baking Powder
pinch Sea Salt
3 tsp Avocado Oil (for the waffle maker)

Notes

Leftovers
Refrigerate in an airtight container for up to three days.
Freeze for up to two months.
Reheat in a toaster or toaster oven.

Serving Size
One serving equals two waffles.

Tuna Salad Plate

5 ingredients · 5 minutes · 1 serving

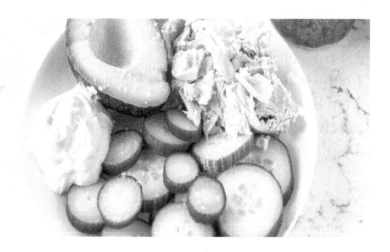

Directions

1. Assemble all the ingredients onto a plate or into a container if on-the-go. Season with salt and enjoy!

Ingredients

1 can Tuna (drained, broken into chunks)

1/2 Avocado (pit removed)

1/4 cup Unsweetened Coconut Yogurt

1/4 Cucumber (sliced)

1/4 tsp Sea Salt

Notes

Leftovers
Refrigerate in an airtight container for up to four days.

More Flavor
Add pepper, paprika and/or lemon juice.

Additional Toppings
Top with sliced green onions, red onion, or red pepper flakes.

Canned Tuna
One can of tuna is equal to 165 grams (5.8 ounces).

No Tuna
Use sardines or salmon instead.

No Coconut Yogurt
Use mayonnaise or Greek yogurt instead.

Turkey & Vegetable Soup

11 ingredients · 50 minutes · 2 servings

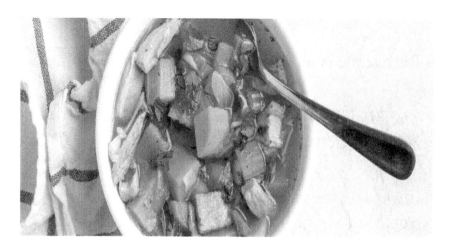

Directions

1. Heat the oil in a large pot over medium heat.

2. Add the onion and cook until it begins to soften, about 5 minutes. Add in the garlic, thyme and salt and continue cooking for one minute more.

3. Add the sweet potato, carrots, celery, and turkey. Stir to combine then add the chicken broth to the pot along with the parsley.

4. Bring soup to a gentle boil then reduce the heat to low and cover with a lid. Simmer for 40 to 45 minutes or until the vegetables are very tender. Season with additional salt if needed.

Ingredients

1 tsp Extra Virgin Olive Oil
1/3 Yellow Onion (chopped)
1 Garlic (clove, minced)
1/3 tsp Dried Thyme
1/3 tsp Sea Salt
1/3 Sweet Potato (peeled, cut into 1/2-inch cubes)
1/3 Carrot (peeled, chopped)
2/3 stalk Celery (chopped)
3 1/2 ozs Turkey Breast, Cooked (roughly chopped)
2 cups Chicken Broth
1/3 cup Parsley (chopped)

Notes

Leftovers
Refrigerate in an airtight container for up to three days.

Serving Size
One serving is approximately 1 1/2 cups of soup.

More Flavor
Add a bay leaf or some red pepper flakes.

No Turkey
Use chicken breast instead.

Whole Wheat Flatbread

1 ingredient · 5 minutes · 1 serving

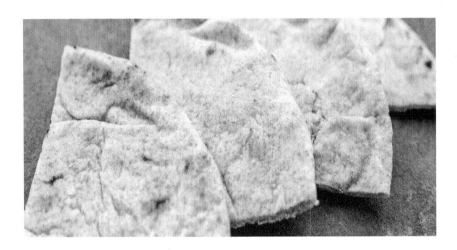

Directions

1. Slice and enjoy at room temperature or warmed up.

Ingredients

1 3/4 ozs Whole Wheat Flatbread

Notes

Serving Size
One serving is equal to approximately 52 grams or one medium-size piece of flatbread.
Warm it up in the toaster, oven, or microwave.
Serve it With Stew or soup, or as a wrap or pizza crust.

Ginger Cilantro Salmon Burgers

7 ingredients · 30 minutes · 1 serving

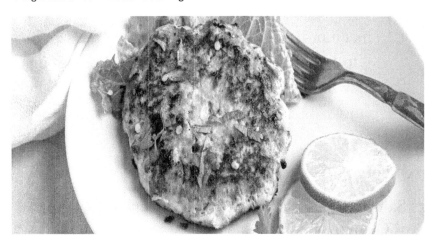

Directions

1. Add the salmon to the bowl of a food processor (including the blade) and place in the freezer for 15 minutes.

2. Meanwhile, in a large mixing bowl combine the cilantro, ginger, coconut aminos, sesame oil and lime juice. Set aside.

3. Remove the food processor bowl from the freezer. Pulse the salmon 4 to 5 times until finely chopped but not a puree. Fold the chopped salmon into the cilantro and ginger mixture.

4. Form the mixture into patties. If it is too wet, refrigerate for 20 minutes to stiffen before

forming into patties.

5. Heat the avocado oil in a large non-stick pan over medium-high heat. Cook the salmon burgers for 4 to 5 minutes per side, or until cooked through and firm to the touch. Serve immediately and enjoy.

Ingredients

4 ozs Salmon Fillet (skinless, cut into 1/2-inch chunks)
2 tbsps Cilantro (finely chopped)
1 1/2 tsps Ginger (peeled and finely grated)
1 tsp Low sodium soy sauce
1/2 tsp Sesame Oil
1/2 tsp Lime Juice
1 1/2 tsps Extra Virgin Olive Oil

Notes

Serving Size
One serving is equal to one salmon burger.

More Flavor
Add minced garlic, honey, lime zest, red pepper flakes or hot sauce to the burger mixture.

Roasted Mini Peppers

3 ingredients · 20 minutes · 1 serving

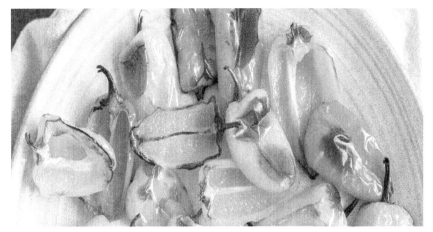

Directions

1. Preheat oven to 400°F (204°C) and line a baking sheet with foil or parchment.

2. Toss mini peppers in the oil and salt, and transfer to the baking sheet cut side down. Roast for 13 to 15 minutes or until slightly charred.

3. Remove from oven and enjoy!

Ingredients

5 1/3 ozs Mini Peppers (halved and seeds removed)
1 tsp Extra Virgin Olive Oil
1/16 tsp Sea Salt

Notes

Leftovers
Refrigerate in an airtight container up to 3 to 5 days.

Greek Chicken Salad

10 ingredients · 45 minutes · 2 servings

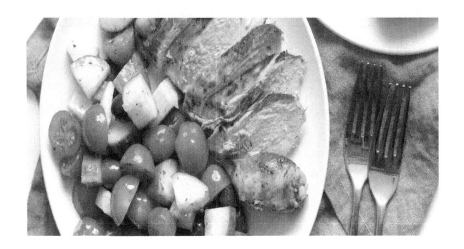

Directions

1. Combine the Greek seasoning, lemon juice, and 1/4 of the olive oil in a shallow bowl or Ziploc bag. Add the chicken breasts and marinate for 20 minutes or overnight.

2. Preheat a grill or skillet over medium heat. Remove chicken from the marinade and cook for 10 to 15 minutes per side, or until chicken is cooked through.

3. While the chicken is cooking, make the salad by combining the cherry tomatoes, cucumbers, red onion, olives, balsamic vinegar, remaining olive oil, salt, and pepper. Mix well.

4. Divide the salad and chicken between plates. Enjoy!

Ingredients

1 tbsp Greek Seasoning
1/2 Lemon (juiced)
2 tbsps Extra Virgin Olive Oil
10 ozs Chicken Breast (boneless, skinless)
1/2 cups Cherry Tomatoes (halved)
1/2 Cucumber (diced)
2 tbsps Red Onion (finely diced)
1/2 cup Pitted Kalamata Olives (chopped)
1 1/2 tbsps Balsamic Vinegar
Sea Salt & Black Pepper (to taste)

Notes

No Greek Seasoning
Use Italian seasoning instead.

Hummus Dippers

4 ingredients · 15 minutes · 1 serving

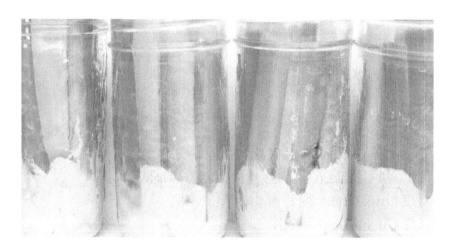

Directions

1. Slice your pepper, carrot, and celery into sticks.

2. Line up 4 small mason jars (we like to use size 250 ml). Fill the bottom of each with ¼ cup hummus. Then place the veggie sticks into the hummus so that they are standing vertically. Seal the jar and place in the fridge until ready to eat.

Ingredients

1/4 Yellow Bell Pepper
1/4 Carrot
1 stalk Celery
1/4 cup Hummus

Notes

Homemade
Make your own hummus! Check out our Sweet Potato Hummus or Green Pea Hummus recipes.

Mix it Up
Substitute in different veggies like cucumber or zucchini.

Bell Peppers with Hummus

2 ingredients · 5 minutes · 1 serving

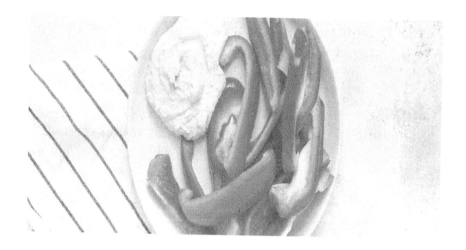

Directions

1. Divide the red bell pepper slices and hummus onto plates and enjoy!

Ingredients

1 Red Bell Pepper (medium, sliced)
1/4 cup Hummus

Notes

Leftovers
Refrigerate in an airtight container for up to three days.

Additional Toppings
Sprinkle paprika over the hummus.

No Red Bell Pepper
Use cucumber slices, celery, carrots, or rice cakes instead

Peach & Almonds

2 ingredients · 5 minutes · 1 serving

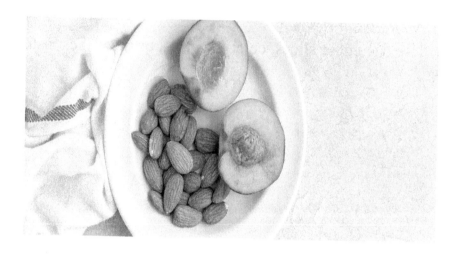

Directions

1. Serve the peach with the almonds and enjoy!

Ingredients

1 Peach (whole, halved or sliced)

1/4 cup Almonds

Notes

Nut-Free
Use pumpkin seeds or sunflower seeds instead.

Sun Butter Pumpkin Protein Balls

6 ingredients · 10 minutes · 1 serving

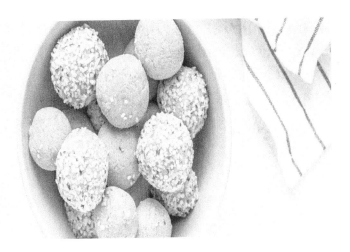

Directions

1. In a mixing bowl, combine the coconut flour, protein powder, sunflower seed butter, pumpkin, and oat milk. Mix well until a firm batter forms. Add more oat milk one tablespoon at a time if the mixture is too dry/crumbly.

2. Form the dough into one-inch balls. Repeat until all the dough is used up. Firmly roll each ball in a small bowl of hemp seeds to form a coating (optional). Store in the fridge or freezer until ready to enjoy.

Ingredients

1 1/4 tsps Coconut Flour
2/3 tsp Vanilla Protein Powder
1 1/4 tsps Sunflower Seed Butter
1 1/4 tsps Pureed Pumpkin
1/3 tsp Oat Milk (unsweetened, plain)
11/4 tsps Hemp Seeds (for coating, optional)

Notes

Leftovers
Refrigerate in an airtight container for up to seven days or freeze if longer.

Serving Size
One serving equals one ball, about one inch in diameter.

More Flavor
Add pumpkin pie spice, and/or vanilla extract.

No Hemp Seeds
Roll in crushed nuts, cocoa powder, pumpkin seeds, or sunflower seeds.

No Sunflower Seed Butter
Use almond butter, tahini, or pumpkin seed butter instead.

Roasted Turkey Breast & Carrots

10 ingredients · 1 hour 5 minutes · 2 servings

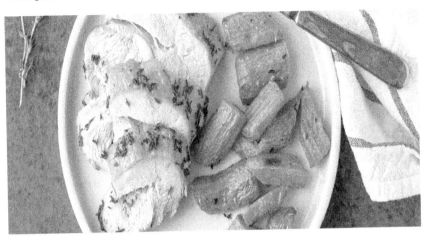

Directions

1. Preheat the oven to 425°F (218°C). Arrange the orange and onion quarters in a large baking dish or a roasting pan.

2. Season the turkey breast on all sides with two-thirds of the salt. Place the seasoned turkey breast on top of the orange and onion in the baking dish.

3. In a small mixing bowl combine half of the oil with the sage, rosemary, and two-thirds of the thyme. Spoon the oil mixture evenly over top of the turkey breast. Add the water to the bottom of the baking dish then bake the turkey breast for 20 minutes.

4. Meanwhile, line a baking sheet with parchment

paper. Place the carrots on the baking sheet and season with the remaining oil and salt.

5. After the turkey has cooked for 20 minutes, reduce the oven to 350°F (176°C). Place the carrots in the oven with the turkey. Continue cooking for 30 to 40 minutes or until the turkey is cooked through, the skin is brown and crispy, and the carrots are cooked. Be sure to add more water to the pan if it evaporates too quickly or if the pan juices start to burn.

6. Let the turkey rest for at least 10 minutes before slicing. Season the roasted carrots with the remaining thyme.

Ingredients

1 1/8 lbs Turkey Breast, Skin on (bone-in)
1/2 Navel Orange (cut into quarters)
1/2 Yellow Onion (cut into quarters)
1/3 tsp Sea Salt (divided)
1 1/2 tbsps Extra Virgin Olive Oil (divided)
1/2 tsp Fresh Sage (finely chopped)
1 1/2 tsps Rosemary (finely chopped)
2 1/4 tsps Thyme (finely chopped, divided)
1/3 cup Water
3 Carrot (medium, peeled, roughly chopped)

House Salad

5 ingredients · 10 minutes · 2 servings

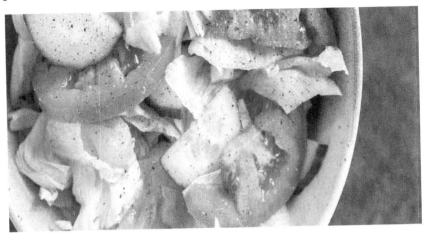

Directions

1. In a small bowl, whisk together the olive oil and vinegar.
2. Add remaining ingredients to a large bowl and drizzle the dressing over top. Toss until well coated. Divide onto plates and enjoy!

Ingredients

2 tbsps Extra Virgin Olive Oil

1 tbsp Red Wine Vinegar

1/4 head Green Lettuce (roughly chopped)

1 Tomato (medium, sliced)

1/2 Cucumber (sliced)

Notes

No Red Wine Vinegar
Use apple cider vinegar or white vinegar instead.

No Lettuce
Use spinach, kale, or mixed greens instead.

More Toppings
Add sliced red onion, bell peppers, celery, and/or avocado.

On-the-Go
Keep dressing in a separate container on the side. Add just before serving.

Steamed White Fish with Tomato & Olive Sauce

9 ingredients · 20 minutes · 1 serving

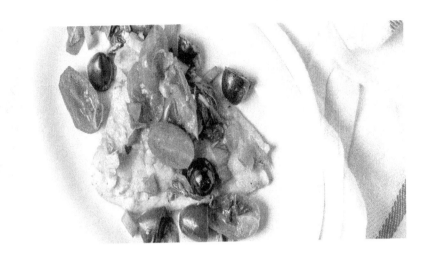

Directions

1. Heat the oil in a medium-sized pan with a lid over medium heat. Season the fish with half of the salt and half of the pepper and set aside.

2. Add the cherry tomatoes to the pan and cook for about five minutes or until the tomatoes have softened and released their juices. Season the tomatoes with the remaining salt and pepper. Add the olives, green onions, basil, and water. Stir to combine, bringing the mixture to a simmer.

3. Place the fish fillets on top of the tomato mixture and cover with a lid. Let the fish steam for 4 to 8 minutes or until the fish is cooked through and

flakes easily.

Ingredients

1/2 tsps Extra Virgin Olive Oil
1/8 tsp Sea Salt (divided)
1/8 tsp Black Pepper (divided)
1/2 cup Cherry Tomatoes (cut in half)
2 tbsps Black Olives (pits removed)
1/2 stalk Green Onion (chopped)
2 tbsps Basil Leaves (chopped)
2 tbsps Water
1 Haddock Fillet or other white fish

Notes

Serving Size
One serving is one fish fillet and approximately 3/4 cup of the tomato & olive sauce.

More Flavor
Add garlic or red pepper flakes. Use low sodium chicken broth instead of water.

Steamed Asparagus

1 ingredient · 10 minutes · 1 serving

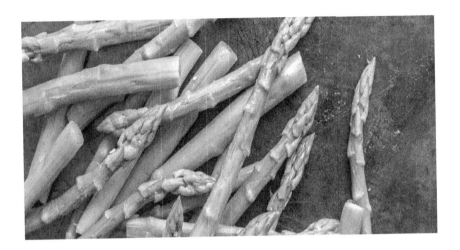

Directions

1. Set the asparagus in a steaming basket over boiling water and cover. Steam for 3 to 5 minutes for thin asparagus, or 6 to 8 minutes for thick asparagus. Enjoy!

Ingredients

1 cup Asparagus (woody ends trimmed, chopped in half)

Notes

Leftovers
Refrigerate in an airtight container up to 5 days.

Serving Size
One serving is equal to approximately one cup of cooked asparagus.

Zucchini Noodles with Salmon

9 ingredients · 20 minutes · 2 servings

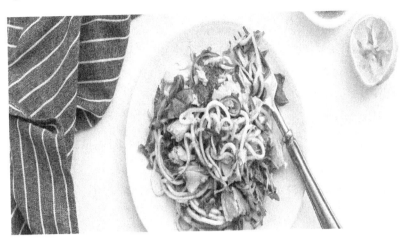

Directions

1. Place the salmon fillet on a baking sheet. Broil on high for 5 to 6 minutes until cooked through and flaky. Let it cool slightly and then slice into bite-sized pieces.

2. In a blender or food processor, add the basil, extra virgin olive oil, garlic, anchovy, lemon juice and sea salt. Blend until smooth.

3. In a pan over medium heat, add the arugula and cook until just wilted. Remove and set aside. Add the zucchini noodles and cook for 3 to 4 minutes. Plate the noodles with the arugula and salmon and drizzle the sauce on top. Serve and enjoy!

Ingredients

6 ozs Salmon Fillet
1 cup Basil Leaves
1/4 cup Extra Virgin Olive Oil
1 Garlic (clove, minced)
1 Anchovy
1/2 tsp Lemon Juice
1/8 tsp Sea Salt
2 cups Arugula
1 Zucchini (large, spiralized into noodles)

Notes

Leftovers
Refrigerate in an airtight container for up to three days. For best results, store the noodles and sauce separately.

Serving Size
One serving is approximately one cup of zucchini noodles and three ounces of salmon fillet.

More Flavor
Add nutritional yeast or chili flakes.

Zucchini Noodles with Salmon

9 ingredients · 20 minutes · 2 servings

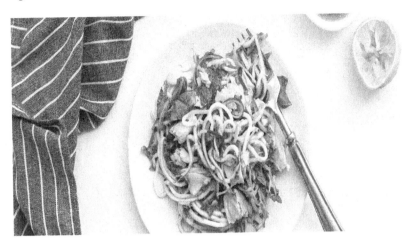

Directions

1. Place the salmon fillet on a baking sheet. Broil on high for 5 to 6 minutes until cooked through and flaky. Let it cool slightly and then slice into bite-sized pieces.

2. In a blender or food processor, add the basil, extra virgin olive oil, garlic, anchovy, lemon juice and sea salt. Blend until smooth.

3. In a pan over medium heat, add the arugula and cook until just wilted. Remove and set aside. Add the zucchini noodles and cook for 3 to 4 minutes. Plate the noodles with the arugula and salmon and drizzle the sauce on top. Serve and enjoy!

Ingredients

6 ozs Salmon Fillet
1 cup Basil Leaves
1/4 cup Extra Virgin Olive Oil
1 Garlic (clove, minced)
1 Anchovy
1/2 tsp Lemon Juice
1/8 tsp Sea Salt
2 cups Arugula
1 Zucchini (large, spiralized into noodles)

Notes

Leftovers
Refrigerate in an airtight container for up to three days. For best results, store the noodles and sauce separately.

Serving Size
One serving is approximately one cup of zucchini noodles and three ounces of salmon fillet.

More Flavor
Add nutritional yeast or chili flakes.

Saffron Chicken Kebab with Salad

10 ingredients · 25 minutes · 2 servings

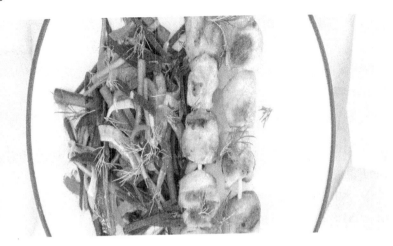

Directions

1. Add the ground saffron to a medium bowl. Add a splash of boiling water and let the saffron bloom for two minutes.

2. Add the cubed chicken thighs to the saffron water. Add 1/2 of the salt and 1/3 of the lemon juice. Mix everything well and thread the chicken cubes onto the skewers.

3. Heat 1/2 of the oil in a heavy bottom pan over medium-high heat. Cook the chicken skewers for about three to four minutes per side.

4. In the meantime, place the cucumbers, beets, and fennel in a medium bowl. Add the remaining salt, lemon juice, oil, and 2/3 of the chopped dill. Mix well.

5. Once the chicken is cooked, divide the skewers and salad onto plates. Sprinkle the remaining dill on top. Enjoy!

Ingredients

1/4 tsp Saffron (ground)
8 ozs Chicken Thighs (boneless, skinless, cut into 1-inch cubes)
1/2 tsp Sea Salt (divided)
1 1/2 tbsps Lemon Juice (divided)
4 Barbecue Skewers
2 tbsps Extra Virgin Olive Oil (divided)
1/2 Cucumber (julienned)
2 Beet (medium, peeled, and julienned)
1/2 bulb Fennel (small, thinly sliced into strips)
2 tbsps Fresh Dill (roughly chopped, divided)

Notes

Serving Size
One serving is equal to approximately two chicken skewers and two cups of salad.

Additional Toppings
Add other fresh herbs such as mint or parsley.

Steamed Green Beans

1 ingredient · 10 minutes · 1 serving

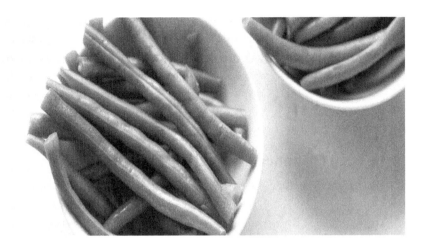

Directions

1. Bring a 1/2-inch of salted water to boil in a large pan. Add green beans, cover, and cook for about 5 to 7 minutes or until desired tenderness is reached.

2. Remove greens beans with a slotted spoon and serve.

Ingredients

1 1/2 cups Green Beans (trimmed, fresh or frozen)

Notes

Use a Steamer Basket
Add green beans to the steamer basket and set over a pot of boiling water. Cover and cook for about 5 minutes or until tender.

More Flavour
Toss the beans in butter, coconut oil or olive oil. Season with your favourite spices.

Serve Them With
Our Roasted Garlic Chicken Thighs and Roasted Sweet Potato Rounds.

Turmeric Beef Stew

14 ingredients · 55 minutes · 2 servings

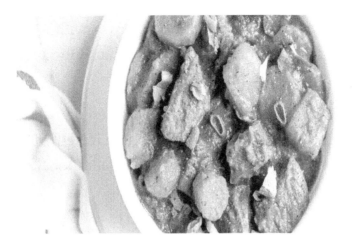

Directions

1. Cut steak into 1-inch cubes. Transfer to a mixing bowl with tapioca flour, salt, and pepper. Toss until the steak is well coated.

2. Heat oil in a Dutch oven or large pot over medium-high heat. Add the beef and brown it on all sides. Remove the beef from the pot and set aside. (Adjust the heat as necessary when browning the steak to prevent the bottom of the pot from burning. You may need to do the browning in batches.)

3. Add the carrots and potatoes to the pot along with the turmeric, coriander, cumin, and ginger. Stir frequently for 2 to 3 minutes. If the spices start sticking to the bottom of the pot add two tablespoons of water to help them along. Add the

browned beef back to the pan.

4. Add the broth to the pot, being sure to scrape the browned bits off the bottom. Cover with a tight-fitting lid, reduce heat to medium-low and let simmer for 20 minutes.

5. Remove the lid and stir in the green onions and cilantro. Continue to simmer uncovered for 10 minutes. Taste and season with additional salt and pepper, if needed.

Ingredients

8 ozs Top Sirloin Steak
1 1/2 tsps Tapioca Flour
1/2 tsp Sea Salt
1/4 tsp Black Pepper
2 1/4 tsps Extra Virgin Olive Oil
1 Carrot (medium, chopped)
1/2 Yellow Potato (large, chopped)
1/2 tsp Turmeric (ground)
1/2 tsp Coriander (ground)
1/2 tsp Cumin (ground)
1/2 tsp Ground Ginger
1 cup Beef Broth
2 stalks Green Onion (green parts only, chopped)
1/4 cup Cilantro (chopped)

Spaghetti Squash Chow Mein

10 ingredients · 1 hour 30 minutes · 1 serving

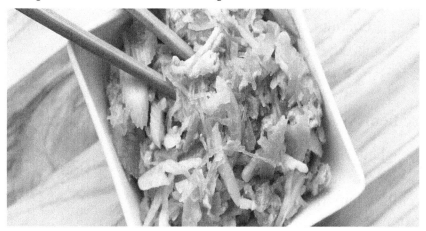

Directions

1. Preheat oven to 350°F (177°C) and slice the spaghetti squash in half. Place cut-side down on a baking sheet and bake in the oven for about 60 minutes or until it can be easily pierced with a fork. When done, remove from oven. Turn over and let cool slightly.

2. While the spaghetti squash is cooling, heat the sesame oil over medium heat in a large skillet or wok. Add the onion, celery, coleslaw mix, garlic, and ginger, stirring to combine. Cover and cook for about 10 minutes, stirring occasionally.

3. In a separate pan, melt the coconut oil and brown the ground chicken.

4. Carefully scoop the flesh out of the spaghetti

squash. Add the spaghetti squash and the chicken to the pan with the sauteed veggies. Pour the coconut aminos over everything and mix well. Divide between bowls. Enjoy!

Ingredients

1/4 Spaghetti Squash
1 1/2 tsps Sesame Oil
1/4 Yellow Onion (medium, diced)
1 stalk Celery (sliced diagonally)
1 cup Coleslaw Mix
3/4 Garlic (cloves, minced)
3/4 tsp Ginger (peeled and grated)
1/3 tsp Coconut Oil
4 ozs Extra Lean Ground Chicken
1 tbsp Tamari

Notes

Vegan and Vegetarian
Replace the ground chicken with scrambled eggs or tofu.

Week Two

Week Two: no sugar, low glycemic, no dairy. Drink plenty of water, water with lemon, spearmint tea, green tea. Only one unsweetened caffeinated drink in the morning.

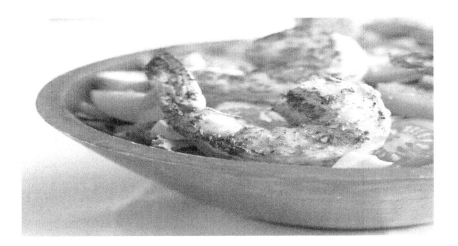

Week Two Meal Plan

	Mon	Tue	Wed	Thu	Fri	Sat	Sun
Breakfast	Detox Green Smoothie	Detox Green Smoothie	Scrambled Eggs with Peppers & Kale	Creamy Blueberry Smoothie	Creamy Blueberry Smoothie	Oatmeal with Raspberries	Spinach & Salsa Omelette
Lunch	Simple Salmon Salad	Creamy Carrot Soup	Creamy Carrot Soup	Chicken Tikka Salad	Chicken Tikka Salad	Grilled Shrimp Salad	Turmeric & Ginger Butternut Squash Stew
	Simple Lentil Flatbread	Turkey & Spinach Wrap	House Salad		Herb & Garlic Quinoa		
	Carrot Sticks	Almonds	Apple	Celery & Hummus	Chopped Bell Peppers	Peach	Pear
Snack	Chopped Bell Peppers		Cherry Tomatoes		Hard Boiled Eggs	Sunbutter Pumpkin Protein Balls	
Dinner	Greek Chicken Salad	Greek Chicken Salad	Sweet Potato Shepherd's Pie	Lemon Cilantro Cod with Peppers	Sweet Potato Shepherd's Pie	Slow Cooker BBQ Pulled Pork	Pan Seared Chicken with Garlicky Cranberry Sauce
			Steamed Asparagus & Zucchini			Steamed Asparagus & Zucchini	Carrots & Broccoli

Detox Green Smoothie

8 ingredients · 10 minutes · 2 servings

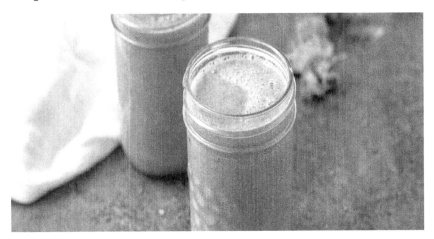

Directions

1. Place all ingredients together in a blender. Blend until smooth. Be patient! No one likes clumps in their smoothies. It may take 1 minute or longer to get a great, smoothie- consistency.

2. Divide between glasses and enjoy!

Ingredients

4 cups Kale Leaves
1 Cucumber (chopped)
1 Lemon (juiced)
2 Pear (peeled and chopped)
1 tbsp Ginger (grated)
1 tbsp Ground Flax Seed

1 1/2 cups Water
5 Ice Cubes

Notes

No Kale
Use spinach.

No Pear
Use apples.

Metabolism Boost
Add 1/4 tsp cayenne pepper.

Scrambled Eggs with Peppers & Kale

5 ingredients · 15 minutes · 1 serving

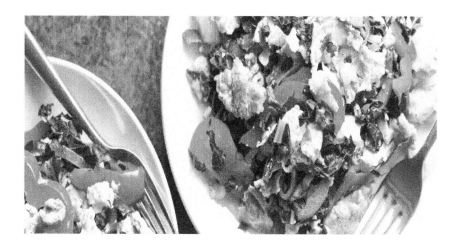

Directions

1. Heat the olive oil in a skillet over medium heat. Add the red bell pepper and kale leaves and sauté until softened, about 5 to 7 minutes.

2. While the veggies are cooking, crack the eggs into a bowl and season with salt and pepper. Beat gently with a fork until well combined.

3. Push the veggies to one side of the pan and pour the beaten eggs into the empty side. Use a spatula to scramble, slowly incorporating the veggies once the eggs are no longer very wet.

4. Divide between plates and enjoy!

Ingredients

3/4 tsp Extra Virgin Olive Oil
1/2 Red Bell Pepper (sliced)
1 cup Kale Leaves (chopped)
3 Egg
Sea Salt & Black Pepper (to taste)

Creamy Blueberry Smoothie

7 ingredients · 5 minutes · 1 serving

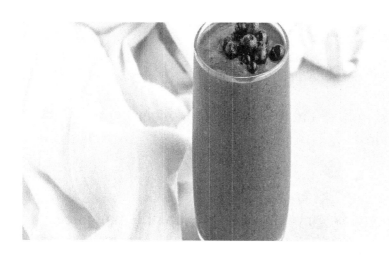

Directions

1. Add all ingredients to a blender and blend until smooth. Pour into a glass and enjoy!

Ingredients

1 cup Frozen Blueberries
1 cup Frozen Cauliflower
1/2 cup Unsweetened Coconut Yogurt
1/4 cup Vanilla Protein Powder
1 tbsp Chia Seeds
1 Lemon (small, juiced)
1 cup Water

Notes

Instead of Protein Powder
Add spinach, or kale

Extra Creamy
Use almond milk or oat milk instead of water.
Add avocado

Lemon
One lemon yields approximately 1/4 cup of lemon juice.

Protein Powder
This recipe was developed and tested using a plant-based protein powder. If using another type of protein powder, note that results may vary.

Oatmeal with Raspberries

4 ingredients · 10 minutes · 1 serving

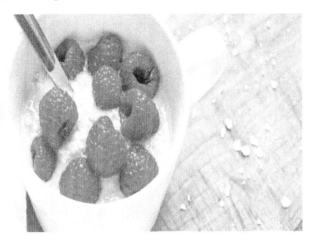

Directions

1. Bring water to a boil in a small saucepan. Add the oats. Reduce to a steady simmer and cook, stirring occasionally for about five minutes or until the oats are tender and most of the water is absorbed.

2. Stir in ground flaxseed.

3. Transfer the cooked oats to a bowl and top with raspberries. Enjoy!

Ingredients

1 cup Water
1/2 cup Oats (quick or rolled)
1 tbsp Ground Flaxseed
1/2 cup Raspberries

Notes

Leftovers
Refrigerate in an airtight container for up to four days.

More Flavor
Add cinnamon, or vanilla extract.

No Raspberries
Top with blueberries, strawberries, peaches, or bananas.

No Stove Top
Cook oats in the microwave instead.

Spinach & Salsa Omelette

5 ingredients · 10 minutes · 1 serving

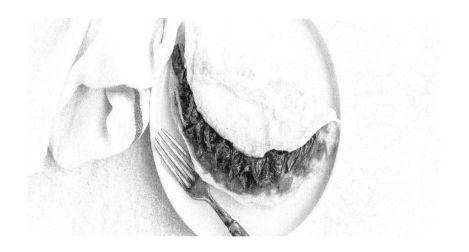

Directions

1. Heat half of the oil in a non-stick pan over medium heat. Add the spinach and cook until tender and wilted. Transfer the cooked spinach to a plate and set aside.

2. Whisk the eggs in a small bowl and season with salt and pepper to taste. Add the remaining oil to the pan. Add the eggs and cook until almost set. Place the salsa and cooked spinach on one half of the omelette and fold the other half over top. Remove from heat and enjoy!

Ingredients

2 tsps Extra Virgin Olive Oil (divided)
2 cups Baby Spinach
3 Eggs
Sea Salt & Black Pepper (to taste)
1/4 cup Salsa

Simple Salmon Salad

6 ingredients · 5 minutes · 1 serving

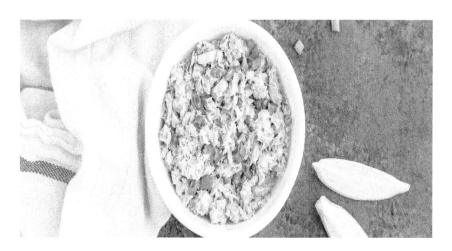

Directions

1. Add the salmon, mayonnaise, and lemon juice to a bowl and mash with a fork until well combined. Stir in the celery and green onion (if using).

2. Season with salt and pepper and additional lemon juice if needed. Enjoy!

Ingredients

4 ozs Canned Wild Salmon (drained)
2 tbsps Mayonnaise
1 1/2 tbsps Lemon Juice
1 stalk Celery (finely chopped, optional)
1 stalk Green Onion (chopped, optional)
Sea Salt & Black Pepper (to taste)

Notes

Leftovers
Refrigerate in an airtight container for up to three days.

More Flavor
Add fresh or dried herbs, mustard, chopped pickles, or garlic.

Serve it With
Use as a filling for sandwiches or wraps, on top of salad greens or cucumber slices.

No Canned Salmon
Use canned tuna or sardines instead.

No Green Onion
Use red onion instead.

No Celery
Use cucumber, bell pepper, or radish.

No Mayonnaise
Use yogurt or mashed avocado instead.

Simple Lentil Flatbread

3 ingredients · 3 hours 30 minutes · 1 serving

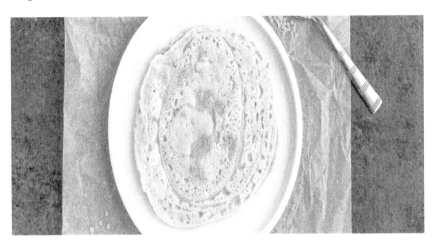

Directions

1. Soak the lentils in 2/3 of the water in the fridge for at least three hours or up to overnight.

2. Drain and rinse the lentils well then transfer to a high-speed blender with the remaining water and the salt. Blend on high speed for about a minute until the batter is smooth and creamy.

3. Heat a non-stick pan over medium heat. Add approximately a 1/4 cup of the batter to the hot pan. Then quickly using a spatula or spoon spread the batter into a circle six to seven inches in diameter.

4. Cook the flatbreads for four to six minutes carefully flipping halfway through (do not overcook). Transfer to a plate or cooling rack

to cool completely. Repeat with the remaining batter.

5. Use the cooked flatbreads for sandwich wraps, tacos, or for dipping. Enjoy!

Ingredients

1 2/3 tbsps Dry Red Lentils

1/3 cup Water (divided)

1/16 tsp Sea Salt

Notes

Leftovers
Store in an airtight container in the refrigerator for up to five days or freeze between pieces of parchment paper for up to three months. Warm in a dry pan for best results.

Serving Size
One serving equals one flatbread.

More Flavor
Add dried herbs and spices to the batter.

Creamy Carrot Soup

11 ingredients · 50 minutes · 2 servings

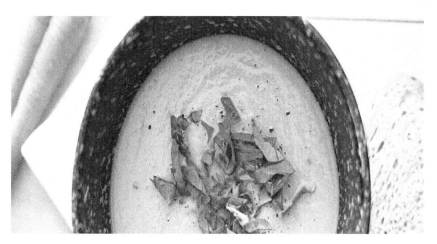

Directions

1. In a large pot, heat olive oil over medium heat. Stir in onion, garlic, carrots, cumin, and turmeric. Season with salt and pepper to taste. Sautee for about 10 minutes or until veggies start to brown.

2. Add in vegetable broth. Cover with lid and let simmer for 30 minutes.

3. After 30 minutes, pour in almond milk and stir well. Transfer soup to a blender to puree. Always be careful to leave a hole for the steam to escape or the lid will pop off while blending. Blend in batches and transfer back to pot. Taste and season with more sea salt and pepper if desired.

4. Ladle soup into bowls. Garnish with chopped

spinach and drizzle with a squeeze of lemon wedge. Serve with a slice of bread for dipping and/or a mixed greens salad.

Ingredients

1 1/2 tsps Extra Virgin Olive Oil
4 Carrot (chopped into 1 inch rounds)
1/2 Sweet Onion (chopped)
1 Garlic (cloves, minced)
1/2 tsp Cumin
1/2 tsp Turmeric
Sea Salt & Black Pepper (to taste)
1 1/2 cups Vegetable Broth
1/2 cup Unsweetened Almond Milk
1/2 Lemon (cut into wedges)
1/2 cup Baby Spinach (chopped)

Notes

Leftovers
Refrigerate in an airtight container for up to four days. Freeze for up to three months.

Serving Size
One serving is roughly 1 1/2 to 2 cups of soup.

Turkey & Spinach Wrap

5 ingredients · 5 minutes · 1 serving

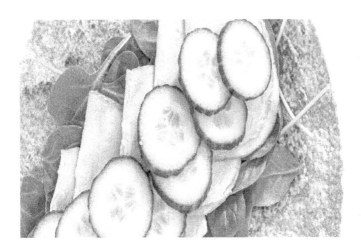

Directions

1. Spread the mustard in the center of the tortilla. Place the spinach, turkey, and cucumber on top. Fold or roll the tortilla around the filling and enjoy!

Ingredients

1 tbsp Dijon Mustard
1 Whole Wheat Tortilla (large)
2 cups Baby Spinach
1/3 ozs Sliced Turkey Breast
1/2 Cucumber (medium, sliced)

Notes

Leftovers
Refrigerate in an airtight container for up to three days.

Gluten-Free
Use a gluten-free tortilla.

Additional Toppings
Add tomatoes, avocado, bell peppers, sliced olives, or sliced red onion.

Chicken Tikka Salad

9 ingredients · 15 minutes · 2 servings

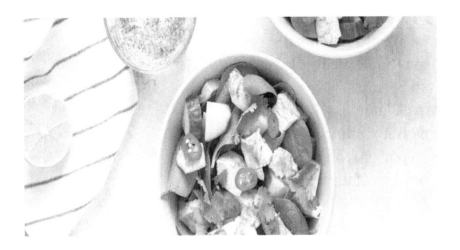

Directions

1. Preheat the oven to 425°F (220°C). Line a baking sheet with foil. Flatten the chicken breast with a mallet or rolling pin to about half-inch thick.

2. Evenly coat the chicken with tikka masala paste and bake for 10 minutes or until cooked through. Slice into cubes.

3. Meanwhile, add the cilantro, lime juice, salt and water in a food processor and blend until well incorporated. Set aside.

4. Divide the spinach, cucumber, chicken, and sliced chili pepper into bowls. Add dressing.

Ingredients

8 ozs Chicken Breast (skinless, boneless)
1 tsp Tikka Masala Paste
1 cup Cilantro (chopped)
2 tbsps Lime Juice
1/8 tsp Sea Salt
3 tbsps Water
3 cups Baby Spinach
1/2 Cucumber (chopped)
1/2 Red Hot Chili Pepper (sliced)

Notes

More Flavor
Add yogurt, turmeric, garlic, oil and/or chutney to the cilantro-lime dressing.

Additional Toppings
Fried mustard and cumin seeds sliced green onion or naan.

Make it Vegan
Use chickpeas, firm tofu, or tempeh instead of chicken.

No Tikka Masala Paste
Use curry paste instead.

Herb & Garlic Quinoa

6 ingredients · 20 minutes · 1 serving

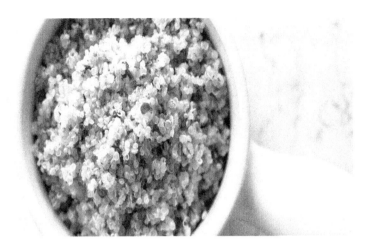

Directions

1. Combine the quinoa and water together in a pot. Place over high heat and bring to a boil. Once boiling, reduce to a simmer and cover. Let simmer for 12 to 15 minutes, or until all water is absorbed. Remove lid, fluff with a fork, and set aside.

2. In a bowl, combine the quinoa, olive oil, parsley, garlic, salt, and pepper. Mix well and enjoy!

Ingredients

1/4 cup Quinoa (dry, uncooked)
1/2 cup Water
1/3 tsp Extra Virgin Olive Oil
1/4 cup Parsley (finely chopped)
1/2 Garlic (cloves, minced)
Sea Salt & Black Pepper (to taste)

Notes

Storage
Refrigerate in an air-tight container up to 4 days or freeze up to 1 month.

Freezer Tip
Squeeze out all the air and flatten your freezer bag to reduce freezer burn and optimize storage space.

Grilled Shrimp Salad

9 ingredients · 25 minutes · 1 serving

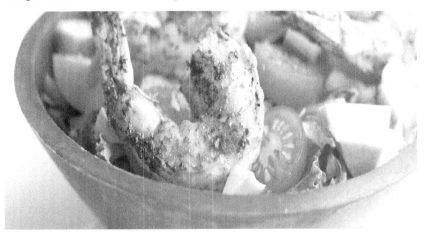

Directions

1. Create dressing by combining the parsley, lime juice, olive oil and chili powder together in a blender or food processor. Process until smooth. Set aside.

2. Throw shrimp in a large Ziplock baggie. Add half of the dressing and shake well to coat. Set the remaining dressing aside.

3. Heat the grill over medium heat. Cook the shrimp for 2 to 3 minutes per side depending on size of shrimp.

4. Divide coleslaw mix between plates and top with avocados, tomatoes, and grilled shrimp. Season with sea salt and pepper to taste. Drizzle remaining dressing over top. Enjoy!

Ingredients

2 tbsps Parsley (chopped and packed)
3/4 Lime (juiced)
1 tbsp Extra Virgin Olive Oil
1/3 tsp Chili Powder
8 ozs Shrimp (raw, peeled, and de-veined)
1 cup Coleslaw Mix
1/4 cup Cherry Tomatoes (halved)
1/4 Avocado (peeled and diced)
Sea Salt & Black Pepper (to taste)

Notes

Vegan & Vegetarian
Use portobello mushrooms instead of shrimp. Marinate and grill the same way.

Turmeric & Ginger Butternut Squash Stew

11 ingredients · 30 minutes · 1 serving

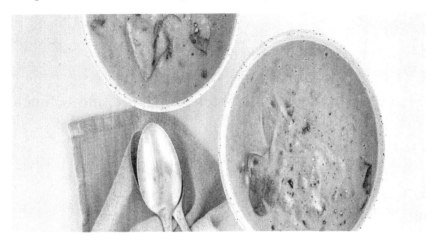

Directions

1. In a large Dutch oven, over medium-low heat, melt the coconut oil. Then add the garlic, ginger, and onion. Sauté for three to five minutes, stirring often, until softened and fragrant.

2. Add in the squash and turmeric and season with salt and pepper. Cook for one minute, stirring often. Pour in the coconut milk, broth, and lentils and stir. Bring to a boil over medium-high heat and then reduce the heat, cover, and simmer for 20 minutes, until lentils and squash are cooked through.

3. Transfer about half of the soup to a blender and carefully purée until smooth. Pour back into the pot and stir in the spinach. Cook until the spinach is wilted. Divide into bowls and serve.

Ingredients

1/3 tsp Coconut Oil
3/4 Garlic (cloves, minced)
3/4 tsp Ginger (freshly grated)
1/4 Yellow Onion (chopped)
1 1/4 cups Butternut Squash (peeled, chopped into 1/2-inch pieces)
1/4 tsp Turmeric (dried)
Sea Salt & Black Pepper (to taste)
1/2 cup Canned Coconut Milk
1 cup Vegetable Broth, Low Sodium
1/4 cup Dry Green Lentils (rinsed)
3/4 cup Baby Spinach

Notes

Serving Size
One serving is equal to approximately two cups of stew.

Sweet Potato Shepherd's Pie

8 ingredients · 35 minutes · 2 servings

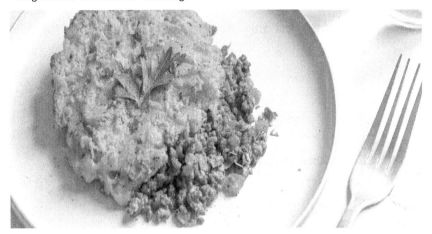

Directions

1. Place the sweet potatoes in a medium pot with just enough water to cover. Bring to a boil and cook until fork-tender, about 10 minutes. Drain the potatoes then mash with the oil and half of the salt. Set aside.

2. Meanwhile, add the beef, onion, carrot, Italian seasoning, garlic powder, and remaining salt to a skillet over medium-high heat. Cook for six to eight minutes until the beef is fully browned and the vegetables have softened. Drain any excess liquid.

3. Set oven broiler to high or 550°F (290°C).

4. Spread the beef filling in an 8X8 baking dish.

Spoon the mashed potatoes on top and smooth them into an even layer. Brush with the remaining oil and broil for 10 to 15 minutes until browned.

Ingredients

1 Sweet Potato (medium, peeled and roughly chopped)
1 1/2 tsps Extra Virgin Olive Oil (divided)
1/2 tsp Sea Salt (divided)
8 ozs Extra Lean Ground Beef
1/2 Yellow Onion (medium, finely chopped)
1/2 Carrot (medium, finely chopped)
1 1/2 tsps Italian Seasoning
1/2 tsp Garlic Powder

Notes

Leftovers

Store in the refrigerator for up to three days or freeze for up to two months.

More Flavor

Add other spices or top with fresh herbs. Add chopped mushrooms or cauliflower to the beef filling.

Steamed Asparagus & Zucchini

2 ingredients · 15 minutes · 1 serving

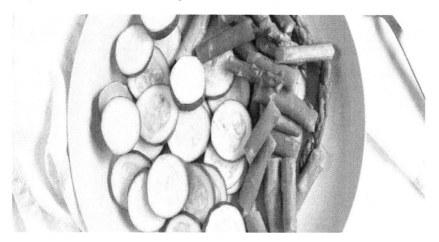

Directions

1. Set the zucchini and asparagus in a steaming basket over boiling water and cover. Steam for 5 to 6 minutes, or until desired texture is reached. Remove from the basket and enjoy!

Ingredients

1/2 Zucchini (sliced)
1/2 cup Asparagus (woody ends trimmed, chopped in quarters)

Notes

Serving Size
One serving is equal to 1 cup of steamed veggies.
More Flavor
Drizzle with olive oil before serving. Add salt and/or pepper.

Lemon Cilantro Cod with Peppers

8 ingredients · 35 minutes · 1 serving

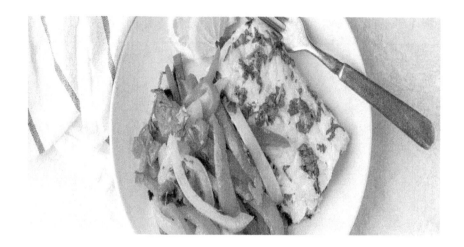

Directions

1. Preheat the oven to 375°F (190°C).

2. In a zipper-lock bag add the lemon juice, 2/3 of the oil, 2/3 of the cilantro and 1/2 of the sea salt. Add the cod and massage the marinade into the fillets. Marinate them for at least 15 minutes or up to an hour.

3. Meanwhile, heat the remaining oil over medium heat. Add the bell peppers and tomato and cook for 8 to 10 minutes or until the peppers are just tender and the tomatoes have released their juices. Stir in the remaining cilantro and season with the remaining salt. Remove from heat.

4. Place cod fillets to a baking dish and transfer the

peppers mixture on top of the cod fillets. Cover the dish with foil, or a tight-fitting lid, and bake for 18 to 20 minutes or until the fish is cooked through and flakes easily.

Ingredients

1 1/2 tbsps Lemon Juice
1 1/2 tbsps Avocado Oil (divided)
1/3 cup Cilantro (finely chopped, divided)
1/4 tsp Sea Salt (divided)
1 Cod Fillet or other white fish
1/4 Red Bell Pepper (sliced)
1/4 Yellow Bell Pepper (sliced)
1/2 Tomato (diced)

Notes

Fillet Size
Each cod fillet is equal to 231 grams or 8 ounces.

More Flavor
Add more herbs like parsley or oregano. Serve with additional lemon wedges.

Slow Cooker BBQ Pulled Pork

10 ingredients · 6 hours · 2 servings

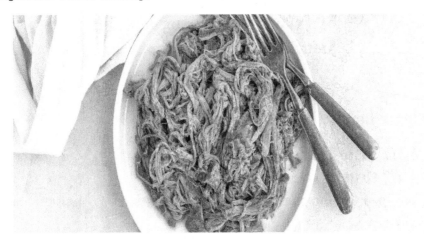

Directions

1. Place pork tenderloin in the slow cooker. Drizzle with olive oil and pour in the broth.

2. In a small bowl, combine sea salt, black pepper, chili powder, paprika, garlic powder, onion powder and cumin. Sprinkle this spice mix over the meat ensuring it is well coated. Cover the slow cooker with a lid and cook on low for 6 to 8 hours, or high for 4 hours or until pork is tender.

3. Once pork is cooked, use two forks to shred it in the slow cooker. Toss it well to coat in the juices and add extra broth if necessary. Let sit for 5 minutes to absorb juices. Toss again and serve. Enjoy!

Ingredients

12 ozs Pork Tenderloin
1 tbsp Extra Virgin Olive Oil
1/2 cup Chicken Broth
1/4 tsp Sea Salt
1/2 tsp Black Pepper
1 1/2 tsps Chili Powder
1 tsp Paprika
1/2 tsp Garlic Powder
1/2 tsp Onion Powder
1/2 tsp Cumin

Notes

Serve it With
Sautéed kale, brown rice, or sweet potato.

Pan Seared Chicken with Garlicky Cranberry Sauce

8 ingredients · 35 minutes · 2 servings

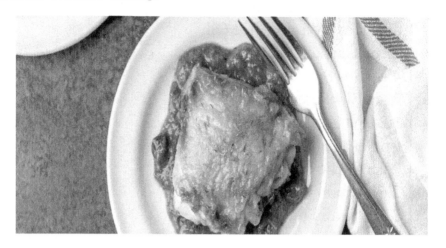

Directions

1. Preheat the oven to 375°F (190°C). Season both sides of the chicken thighs with the salt.

2. In a large cast-iron skillet, or another oven-safe pan, heat the oil over medium-high heat. Brown the seasoned chicken thighs starting with skin-side down for 5 to 7 minutes then flip and brown the other side for another 2 to 3 minutes.

3. Add the frozen cranberries and half of the broth to the pan. Transfer to the oven and bake for 12 to 15 minutes or until the chicken is cooked through. Remove the chicken, place it on a plate and keep warm.

4. Place the pan with the cranberries over medium

heat and add the garlic, thyme, coconut aminos and the remaining stock and stir to combine. Bring the sauce to a gentle boil and let it simmer until the sauce has thickened, about 8 minutes. Season with additional salt if needed.

Ingredients

12 ozs Chicken Thighs (bone-in, skin on)
1/8 tsp Sea Salt
3/4 tsp Extra Virgin Olive Oil
1/4 cup Frozen Cranberries
1/2 cup Chicken Broth (divided)
1 Garlic (clove, minced)
1/4 tsp Dried Thyme
1 1/2 tsps Low Sodium Soy Sauce

Notes

Make it a Meal
Serve with roasted veggies and quinoa or rice.

Carrots & Broccoli

3 ingredients · 15 minutes · 1 serving

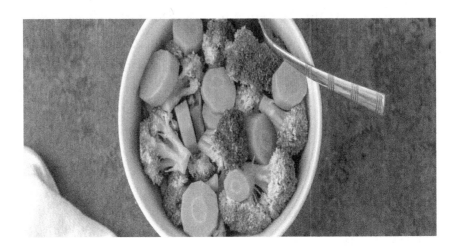

Directions

1. Bring a pot of water to a boil and add the salt, if using.

2. Add the carrots and cook for 5 minutes then add the broccoli to the pot and continue cooking for about 5 minutes more or until the vegetables are tender. Drain and serve.

Ingredients

1/8 tsp Sea Salt (optional)

1 Carrot (peeled, chopped)

1 cup Broccoli (cut into florets)

Week Three

Week Three: No sugar, low glycemic, no dairy, gluten free. Drink plenty of water, spearmint tea, green tea, water with lemon. Only one caffeinated drink in the morning. You can substitute kale for spinach.

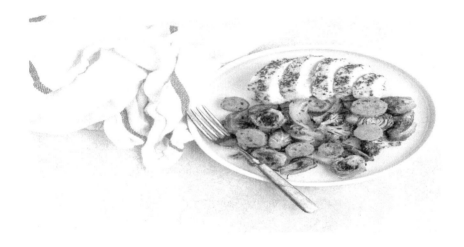

Week Three Meal Plan

	Mon	Tue	Wed	Thu	Fri	Sat	Sun
Breakfast	Cinnamon Pear Oatmeal	Scrambled Eggs with Peppers & Kale	Kiwi Lime Smoothie	Black Bean Egg White Omelette	Detox Green Smoothie	Fluffy Kale & Mushroom Egg White Omelette	Asian Veggie Omelette
Lunch	Slow Cooker Cod & Sea Veggie Soup	Sheet Pan Roasted Chicken & Veggies	Spicy Shrimp, Quinoa & Spinach	Simple Salmon Salad	Rosemary Lemon Chicken Skillet	Okra & Beef Stew	Brussels Sprouts Slaw with Chicken
Snack 2	Celery with Peanut Butter	Brazil Nuts & Blueberries	Hard Boiled Eggs / Chopped Bell Peppers	Apple	Almonds & Raspberries	Pear & Walnuts	Blueberries
Dinner	Sheet Pan Roasted Chicken & Veggies	Spicy Shrimp, Quinoa & Spinach	Salmon with Rice & Greens	Rosemary Lemon Chicken Skillet / House Salad	Okra & Beef Stew	Brussels Sprouts Slaw with Chicken	Lemony Cod & Herbed Rice / House Salad

Cinnamon Pear Oatmeal

6 ingredients · 15 minutes · 1 serving

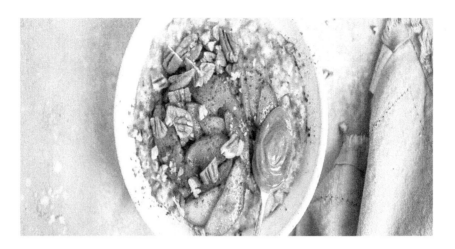

Directions

1. Heat a small non-stick pan over medium heat. Once warm, add the pear and cinnamon. Cook, stirring often until softened and cooked through, about 5 to 7 minutes. Remove the pears and set aside.

2. Meanwhile, add the oats and water to a small saucepan and cook over medium heat, stirring often until gently boiling. Reduce the heat and simmer until cooked through, about 5 to 7 minutes.

3. Add the oats to a bowl and top with pears. Add the pecans and almond butter, if using. Enjoy!

Ingredients

1/2 Pear (sliced)
1/8 tsp Cinnamon 1/2 cup Oats (rolled)
1 cup Water
2 tbsps Pecans (roughly chopped, optional) or pumpkin seeds
1 tbsp Almond Butter (optional)

Notes

More Flavor
Add a splash of oat milk and/or vanilla.

Kiwi Lime Smoothie

4 ingredients · 5 minutes · 1 serving

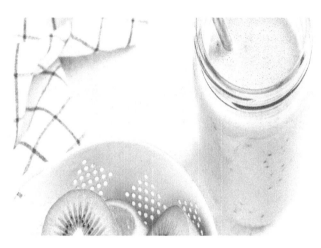

Directions

1. Place all ingredients in a blender and blend until smooth. Pour into a glass and enjoy!

Ingredients

1 cup Unsweetened Almond Milk
2 Kiwi (peeled, halved)
1 Lime (juiced)
1/4 cup Vanilla Protein Powder

Notes

Nut-Free
Use coconut or oat milk instead of almond milk.

Additional Toppings
Add spinach, avocado, kale, ginger, or cucumber to your smoothie.

Protein Powder
This recipe was developed and tested using a plant-based protein powder. If using another type of protein powder, note that results may vary.

Black Bean Egg White Omelette

7 ingredients · 10 minutes · 2 servings

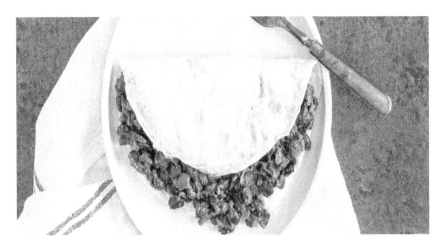

Directions

1. Add the black beans, salsa, and cumin to a pot over medium. Cook for three to five minutes or until the salsa is simmering and the black beans have warmed through. Add the spinach and cook until wilted. If the sauce becomes too thick add a splash of water. Season with salt and pepper and set aside.

2. Heat the oil in a non-stick pan over medium heat. Season the egg whites with salt and pepper then pour into the pan and cook until almost set. Place the black beans on one half of the omelette and fold the other half over top.

Ingredients

1 cup Black Beans (cooked and rinsed)
1/2 cup Salsa
1 tsp Cumin (optional)
1 cup Baby Spinach (chopped)
 Sea Salt & Black Pepper (to taste)
1 tsp Extra Virgin Olive Oil
1 cup Egg Whites

Notes

Leftovers
Refrigerate in an airtight container for up to three days.

More Flavor
Add red pepper flakes, cilantro, lime juice, or taco seasoning to the black beans.

Additional Toppings
Avocado slices, hot sauce, or more salsa.

No Spinach
Use another leafy green, like kale or arugula.

Fluffy Kale & Mushroom Egg White Omelette

7 ingredients · 10 minutes · 2 servings

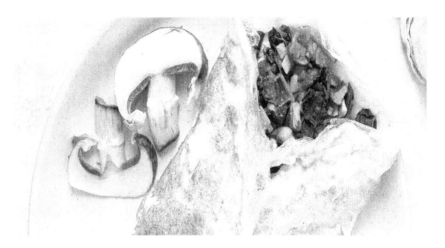

Directions

1. In a large non-stick pan, heat 1/3 of the water over medium heat. Cook the kale, mushrooms, nutritional yeast, garlic powder, and salt until soft, about two minutes. Set aside.

2. Add the remaining water to the same pan and bring to a simmer over medium to medium-high heat. Add the egg whites and cook until fluffy and slightly firm, about five minutes. Rotate the pan as needed to help spread and evenly cook the egg whites. Using a heat-safe spatula, gently scrape down the sides and transfer to a plate.

3. Arrange the kale and mushrooms down the middle of the omelette. Fold the sides of the

omelette towards the center and enjoy!

Ingredients

1/2 cups Water (divided)
2 cups Kale Leaves (tough stems removed, chopped)
8 Cremini Mushrooms (diced)
2 tsps Nutritional Yeast
1/4 tsp Garlic Powder
1/4 tsp Sea Salt
2 cups Egg Whites

Notes

More Flavor

Sauté the kale and mushrooms with olive oil instead of water. Add a squeeze of lemon juice overtop.

No Nutritional Yeast
Use parmesan, feta, vegan cheese, or omit completely.

No Non-Stick Pan
Use your choice of oil as needed.

Asian Veggie Omelette

6 ingredients · 20 minutes · 1 serving

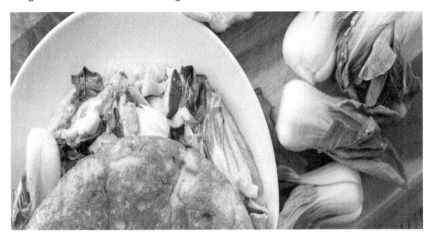

Directions

1. Heat olive oil in a medium-sized frying pan over medium heat. Sauté the Bok choy for 2 minutes. Add mushrooms and cook for 2-3 more minutes or until all veggies are soft. Transfer the veggies to a bowl and set aside.

2. In a bowl, whisk together eggs, tamari, and green onion.

3. Pour the egg mixture into the same pan over medium heat and let cook until almost set. Place the mushrooms and Bok choy on one half of the omelette and fold the other half over top. Remove from heat and season with sea salt and black pepper to taste. Enjoy!

Ingredients

1/2 tsps Olive Oil
1/2 cup Shiitake Mushrooms (sliced)
1 cup Bok Choy (sliced into quarters)
3 Eggs
1/4 tsps Tamari
2 stalks Green Onion (sliced)

Notes

Make it Fluffy
Whisk unsweetened almond milk into your egg mixture.

Mix it Up
Use up whatever vegetables you have on hand. Red onion, bell peppers or baby spinach work well

Likes it Spicy
Serve with hot sauce.

Slow Cooker Cod & Sea Veggie Soup

9 ingredients · 6 hours · 1 serving

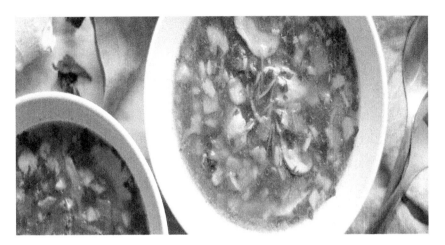

Directions

1. Heat the coconut oil in a frying pan over medium heat. Add the onion and mushrooms. Sauté for about 3 minutes or until onions are translucent. Add garlic and ginger. Cook for a 1 to 2 minutes until fragrant.

2. Transfer the contents of the pan to your slow cooker. Add the dulse (ripped into bite-sized pieces), diced sweet potato, cod, and broth. Do not add salt, as the dulse is naturally very salty and should flavour the soup.

3. Cook on high for 4 hours, or low for 6 to 8 hours. Taste, and add sea salt if necessary.

4. Divide between bowls and enjoy!

Ingredients

2 1/4 tsps Coconut Oil
1/4 Yellow Onion (medium, diced)
1 cup Mushrooms (sliced)
3/4 Garlic (cloves, minced)
1 1/2 tsps Ginger (peeled and grated)
1/3 oz Dulse (torn apart into small pieces)
1/2 Sweet Potato (medium, diced)
1 Cod Fillet (cubed)
2 cups Vegetable Broth (or bone broth)

Notes

Leftovers
Store in an airtight container up to 3 days or freeze.

Fillet Size
One fillet is equal to 231 grams or 8 ounces.

Sheet Pan Roasted Chicken & Veggies

9 ingredients · 30 minutes · 2 servings

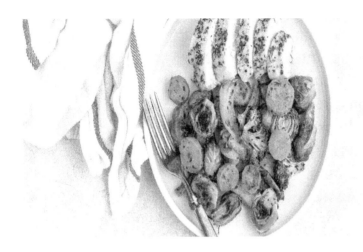

Directions

1. Preheat the oven to 400°F (204°C) and line a baking sheet with parchment paper.

2. Add the veggies and the chicken to the baking sheeting then drizzle with the oil and season with the Italian seasoning, garlic powder, and salt.

3. Bake for 25 minutes or until the chicken is cooked through and the veggies are tender. Season with additional salt if needed.

Ingredients

2 cups Brussels Sprouts (halved or quartered)
1 cup Broccoli (cut into small florets)
1 Carrot (peeled, thinly sliced)
1 Yellow Onion (medium, cut into wedges)
8 ozs Chicken Breast
1 tbsp Extra Virgin Olive Oil
1 tsp Italian Seasoning
1/2 tsp Garlic Powder
1/4 tsp Sea Salt

Notes

Leftovers
Refrigerate in an airtight container for up to three days.

No Chicken Breast
Use chicken thighs or drumsticks instead.

Serve it With
Cauliflower rice, quinoa, brown rice, roasted potatoes, or mashed sweet potato.

Spicy Shrimp, Quinoa & Spinach

10 ingredients · 20 minutes · 2 servings

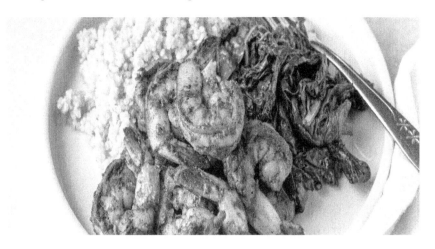

Directions

1. Combine the quinoa and water in a saucepan. Place over high heat and bring to a boil. Once boiling, reduce the heat to a simmer and cover with a lid. Let it simmer for 12 minutes, or until all the water is absorbed and the quinoa is tender.

2. In a mixing bowl combine the oil, garlic, chili powder, cumin, cayenne, and sea salt. Add the shrimp to the bowl and toss to coat evenly in the marinade.

3. Heat a large non-stick pan over medium-high heat. Add the shrimp and the marinade to the hot pan and cook for 4 to 5 minutes stirring often until the shrimp are cooked through. Season with

additional salt if needed. Transfer the shrimp to a dish.

4. Reduce the heat to medium and to the same skillet add the remaining oil. Add the baby spinach and sauté just until wilted.

Ingredients

1/4 cup Quinoa (uncooked)
1/2 cup Water
1 tbsp Extra Virgin Olive Oil (divided)
1/2 Garlic (clove, minced)
1 tsp Chili Powder
1/2 tsp Cumin
1/16 tsp Cayenne Pepper
1/16 tsp Sea Salt
8 ozs Shrimp (raw, peeled, deveined)
6 cups Baby Spinach

Notes

More Flavor

Add more cayenne, red pepper flakes or black pepper to the shrimp marinade for more spice. Serve with lime wedges.

Salmon with Rice & Greens

8 ingredients · 30 minutes · 2 servings

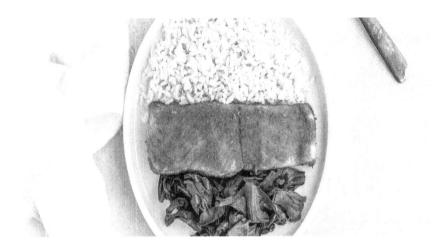

Directions

1. Preheat the oven to 400°F (204°C) and line a baking sheet with parchment paper.

2. Cook the rice according to package directions.

3. In a small bowl combine the paprika, cumin, oregano, and salt. Generously coat all sides of the salmon with the spice blend. Place the salmon on the prepared baking sheet and bake for 16 to 18 minutes or until the salmon is cooked through.

4. Meanwhile, heat a pan over medium heat. Add the water and Swiss chard and cook for three to five minutes, or until the chard is wilted and tender.

5. To serve, divide the rice, salmon and greens between plates or meal prep containers.

Ingredients

1/2 cup Brown Rice (uncooked)
1 tsp Paprika
3/4 tsp Cumin
1/2 tsp Oregano (dried)
1/4 tsp Sea Salt
12 ozs Salmon Fillet
2 tbsps Water
4 cups Swiss Chard (chopped)

Notes

No Swiss Chard
Use spinach or kale instead.

No Brown Rice
Use wild rice, quinoa, or cauliflower rice instead.

Rosemary Lemon Chicken Skillet

8 ingredients · 50 minutes · 2 servings

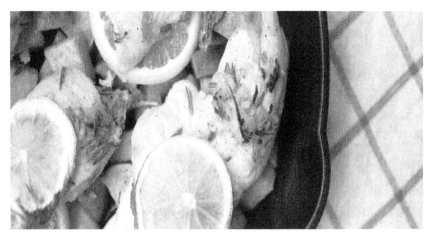

Directions

1. Make the chicken marinade by combining rosemary, lemon juice, lemon zest, half of your olive oil, garlic, and salt in a bowl. Mix well. Add chicken breast halves and marinade to a zip loc bag and seal. Shake and set aside while you prep the rest.

2. Preheat oven to 425°F (218°C).

3. Heat remaining olive oil over medium-high heat in a large cast iron skillet. Add sweet potatoes and cook until potatoes soften (about 5 minutes) and remove from heat.

4. Arrange chicken breast halves and lemon slices over the sweet potatoes in the cast iron skillet. Pour the remaining marinade from the Ziplock

bag over the sweet potatoes. Bake uncovered for about 40 to 45 minutes, or until chicken and potatoes are fully cooked.

5. Remove from oven and plate sweet potato and chicken over a bed of spinach. Enjoy!

Ingredients

8 ozs Chicken Breast (sliced in half)
1 tbsp Rosemary (chopped)
1 Lemon (divided, 1/2 sliced into rounds, 1/2 zested and juiced)
1 1/2 tbsps Extra Virgin Olive Oil (divided)
1 1/2 Garlic (cloves, minced)
1/2 tsp Sea Salt
1 Sweet Potato (cubed)
2 cups Baby Spinach

Notes

Vegetarian
Use cauliflower steaks instead of chicken.

Leftovers
Store in the fridge for up to three days.

Okra & Beef Stew

10 ingredients · 40 minutes · 2 servings

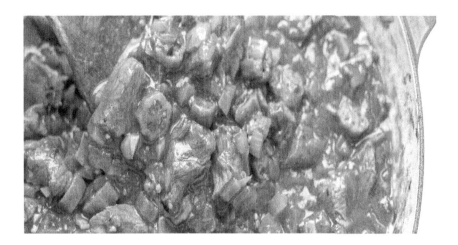

Directions

1. In a large pan over medium-high heat, heat a splash of the water and cook the beef for about eight minutes, flipping halfway. Set aside the beef.

2. In the same pan, heat a few more tablespoons of the water and cook the garlic, onion, and cilantro for about two minutes. Stir in the Lebanese seven spice and okra. Cook until the okra is tender, about 10 minutes. Add more water as needed to prevent sticking.

3. Stir in the cooked beef, tomato paste, tomatoes, sea salt, and the remaining water. Lower the heat to a simmer, cover with a lid, and cook for about

15 minutes or until your desired consistency is reached.

Ingredients

2 3/4 cups Water
10 2/3 ozs Stewing Beef (cubed)
2 Garlic (cloves, minced)
2/3 Yellow Onion (small, diced)
2 2/3 tbsps Cilantro (chopped)
1 tsp Lebanese 7 Spice Blend
2 2/3 cups Okra (trimmed, sliced)
1/3 cup Tomato Paste
1 1/3 Tomato (chopped)
1/3 tsp Sea Salt

Notes

Serving Size
One serving equals approximately 2 1/2 cups.

More Flavor
Cook the beef, onions, and garlic in oil instead of water.

Make it Vegan
Use beans or add more veggies instead of beef.

Brussels Sprouts Slaw with Chicken

9 ingredients · 20 minutes · 2 servings

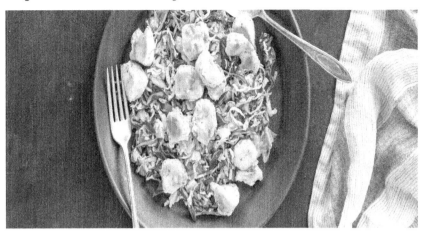

Directions

1. Add the cubed chicken to a small bowl with the oregano, garlic powder and half the salt. Toss to combine.

2. Heat a skillet over medium heat and add 1/3 of the oil. Once hot, add the chicken and cook for 10 to 12 minutes or until cooked through. Remove and set aside.

3. Add the brussels sprouts and cabbage to a bowl. Add the lemon juice, coconut aminos, remaining oil and remaining salt. Mix well with your hands to combine.

4. Divide the slaw evenly between plates. Top with chicken and enjoy!

Ingredients

8 ozs Chicken Breast (cut into cubes)
1/4 tsp Oregano (dried)
1/8 tsp Garlic Powder
1/4 tsp Sea Salt (divided)
1 1/2 tbsps Extra Virgin Olive Oil (divided)
3 cups Brussels Sprouts (shredded)
2 cups Purple Cabbage (sliced thin)
1 1/2 tbsps Lemon Juice
1 tsp Tamari

Notes

More Flavor
Add additional spices and/or herbs to the dressing or chicken.

Additional Toppings
Sliced onion, avocado, slivered almonds, sesame, or sunflower seeds.

Make it Vegan
Omit the chicken and use grilled tofu.

Lemony Cod & Herbed Rice

9 ingredients · 35 minutes · 1 serving

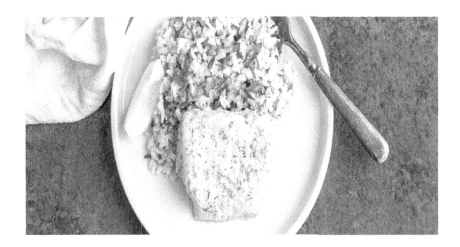

Directions

1. To a shallow bowl or zipper-lock bag, add the Dijon mustard, lemon juice, dill, half of the salt, and half of the garlic powder. Mix to combine. Add the cod fillets to the marinade and ensure the fish is well coated in the sauce and marinate for at least 15 minutes.

2. Meanwhile, add the rice, water, and the remaining salt and garlic powder to a pot. Bring to a boil then reduce the heat, cover, and simmer for about 30 minutes or until the liquid is absorbed and the rice is tender. Stir in the parsley.

3. While the rice cooks, preheat the oven to 375°F

(190ºC).

4. Transfer the fillets and any excess marinade to a baking dish and cover with a lid or foil. Bake for 14 to 16 minutes or until the fish is flakey and cooked through. (Cooking time may vary depending on the thickness of the fillets.) To serve, divide the fish and rice between plates and enjoy!

Ingredients

1 1/2 tsps Dijon Mustard
1 tbsp Lemon Juice
1/8 tsp Dried Dill
1/8 tsp Sea Salt (divided)
1/8 tsp Garlic Powder (divided)
1 Cod Fillet or other white fish
1/4 cup Brown Rice
1/2 cup Water
1 1/2 tsps Parsley (finely chopped)

Week Four

Week Four: No sugar, low glycemic, no dairy, gluten free, corn free. Kale can be switched for spinach or other leafy greens.

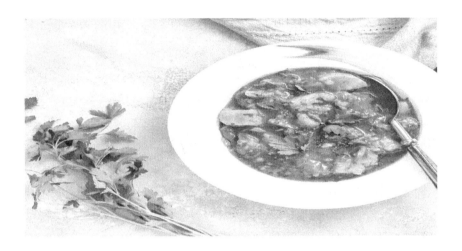

Week Four Meal Plan

MON	TUES	WED	THURS	FRI	SAT	SUN
Cinnamon Protein Oats	Spinach & Salsa Omelette	Berry Avocado Smoothie	Blueberry Protein Smoothie Mushroom & Tofu Scramble	Quinoa & Egg Breakfast Plate	Pear & Kale Protein Smoothie	Pear & Kale Protein Smoothie Grain-Free Flax Bread
Chicken, Asparagus & Sweet Potato	Shrimp Zoodle Stir Fry	Spicy Edamame Fried Cauliflower Rice	Zucchini Noodles with Cauliflower Alfredo	One Pan Steak Fajitas	Seared Cod & Lemon White Beans	Pressure Cooker Beef & Veggie Stew
Apple with Almond Butter	Raspberries	Hard Boiled Eggs	Carrot Sticks Celery & Hummus	Blackberries	Spinach & Sausage Egg Muffins	Spinach & Sausage Egg Muffins
Shrimp Zoodle Stir Fry	Spicy Edamame Fried Cauliflower Rice	Zucchini Noodles with Cauliflower Alfredo	One Pan Steak Fajitas	Seared Cod & Lemon White Beans	Pressure Cooker Beef & Veggie Stew	Spicy Shrimp, Quinoa & Spinach

Cinnamon Protein Oats

4 ingredients · 10 minutes · 1 serving

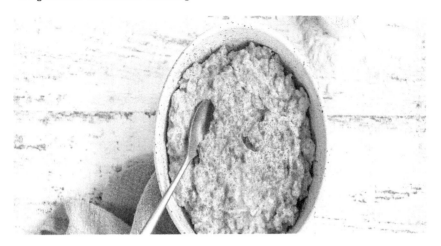

Directions

1. Bring water to a boil in a small saucepan. Add the oats. Reduce to a steady simmer and cook, stirring occasionally for about seven to eight minutes or until oats are tender and most of the water is absorbed. Stir in the protein powder and cinnamon.

2. Transfer the cooked oats to a bowl and enjoy!

Ingredients

1 cup Water
1/2 cup Oats
1/4 cup Vanilla Protein Powder
1/8 tsp Cinnamon

Notes

Leftovers
Refrigerate in an airtight container for up to four days.

Additional Toppings
Berries, fruit, nuts, or seeds.

Berry Avocado Smoothie

7 ingredients · 5 minutes · 1 serving

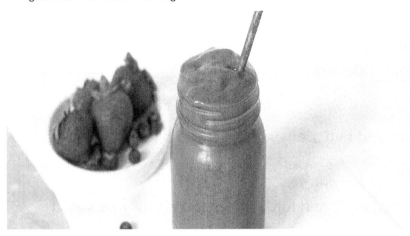

Directions

1.   Place all ingredients in your blender and blend until smooth. Pour into a glass and enjoy!

Ingredients

1 cup Plain Coconut Milk (unsweetened, from the box)
1/2 Zucchini (chopped, frozen)
1/4 cup Frozen Cauliflower
1/2 cup Frozen Berries
1/4 Avocado
tbsp Chia Seeds
1/4 cup Vanilla Protein Powder

Notes

No Chia Seeds
Use flax seeds instead.

No Avocado
Use almond butter or sunflower seed butter instead.

Additional Toppings
Serve in a bowl and top with shredded coconut, sliced banana, or berries.

Protein Powder
This recipe was developed and tested using a plant-based protein powder.

Blueberry Protein Smoothie

5 ingredients · 5 minutes · 2 servings

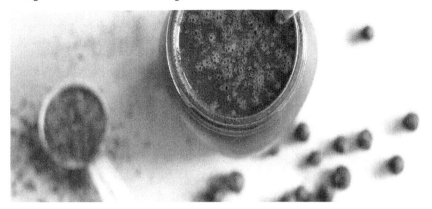

Directions

1. Place all ingredients in your blender and blend until smooth. Pour into a glass and enjoy!

Ingredients

1/2 cup Vanilla Protein Powder
2 tbsps Ground Flax Seed
2 cups Frozen Blueberries
2 cups Baby Spinach
2 cups Water (cold)

Notes

No Frozen Blueberries
Use fresh berries with 1 cup of ice and blend for a cold drink.

No Protein Powder
Use hemp seeds instead.

Mushroom & Tofu Scramble

6 ingredients · 10 minutes · 2 servings

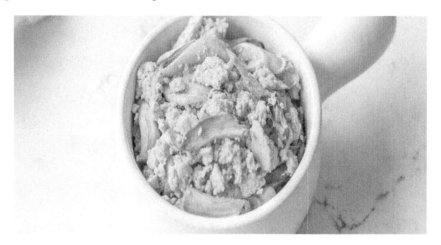

Directions

1. Heat a large skillet over medium heat for 2 minutes. Add the mushrooms and sauté for 3 to 5 minutes, stirring often. Add half of the broth if they begin to stick. Transfer to a plate.

2. Add the remainder of the broth, crumbled tofu, nutritional yeast, turmeric and salt to the skillet. Stir and cook until the tofu is warmed through.

3. Return the mushrooms to the skillet and combine with the tofu. Divide onto plates or containers if on-the-go. Enjoy!

Ingredients

1/2 cup Oyster Mushrooms (sliced)
2 2/3 tbsps Vegetable Broth (divided)
8 ozs Tofu (extra firm, drained, crumbled)
2 tsps Nutritional Yeast
1/8 tsp Turmeric
1/8 tsp Sea Salt

Notes

Leftovers
Refrigerate in an airtight container for up to five days.

Serving Size
Each serving equals approximately 1.5 cups.

More Flavor
Add your choice of spices and/or herbs.

Additional Toppings
Top with sliced green onions, spinach, mixed greens, peppers, or avocado slices.

No Vegetable Broth
Use water instead.

Quinoa & Egg Breakfast Plate

7 ingredients · 20 minutes · 1 serving

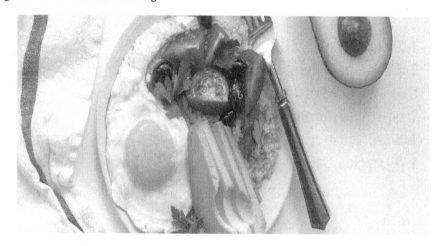

Directions

1. Cook the quinoa according to package directions. Let it cool slightly.

2. In a pan over medium heat, cook the egg until your whites are set and the yolks are your desired doneness.

3. Place the quinoa on a plate, and top with the egg, tomatoes, olives, avocado, and parsley. Season with sea salt and enjoy!

Ingredients

1/4 cup Quinoa (uncooked, rinsed)
1 Egg
2 Tomato (small, chopped)

2 tbsps Pitted Kalamata Olives
1/2 Avocado (sliced)
tbsp Parsley (chopped)
1/8 tsp Sea Salt

Notes

Leftovers
Refrigerate in an airtight container for up to three days.

More Flavor
Cook your quinoa in broth instead of water. Add chili flakes or hot sauce before serving.

Make it Vegan
Omit the egg and serve with tofu or chickpeas instead.

Meal Prep
Make a large batch of quinoa and/or hard-boiled eggs to save time.

Pear & Kale Protein Smoothie

4 ingredients · 5 minutes · 2 servings

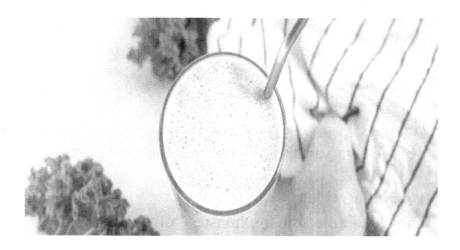

Directions

1. Add all ingredients into a blender and blend until smooth. Divide into glasses and enjoy!

Ingredients

1/2 cups Water (cold)
2 cups Kale Leaves
1 Pear (stem and seeds removed, chopped)
1/2 cup Vanilla Protein Powder
1 tbsp Ground Flaxseed

Notes

Leftovers
Best enjoyed immediately. Refrigerate in an airtight jar for up to two days.

No Kale
Use spinach instead.

No Protein Powder
Omit, or add a few spoonfuls of hemp seeds instead.

Grain-Free Flax Bread

6 ingredients · 1 hour · 1 serving

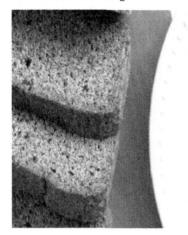 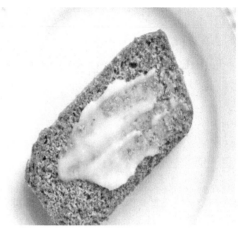

Directions

1. Preheat oven to 350°F (177°C). Grease the inside of a loaf pan or line it with parchment paper.

2. In a medium size bowl, mix together flax, baking powder, and salt. Use a whisk to stir until well combined.

3. In another bowl, beat eggs with a whisk for 30 to 60 seconds. Add water and coconut oil, mixing until combined.

4. Add wet ingredients to dry and stir until combined. Let the batter sit for 1 to 2 minutes to thicken slightly.

5. Pour batter into loaf pan and smooth out the top with a spoon. Bake for about 50 minutes,

or until the top feels set and the loaf is browned.

6. Once cooled, slice and store in the fridge or freezer.

Ingredients

3 1/4 tbsps Ground Flax Seed
1/3 tsp Baking Powder
1/16 tsp Sea Salt
1/2 Egg (room temp)
2 1/3 tsps Water (room temp)
1 1/2 tsps Coconut Oil (melted)

Notes

Leftovers
Refrigerate in an airtight container or food wrap for up to five days. Freeze for up to two months.

Serving Size
One serving is one slice of bread.

Chicken, Asparagus & Sweet Potato

4 ingredients · 30 minutes · 1 serving

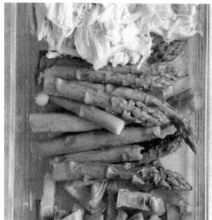
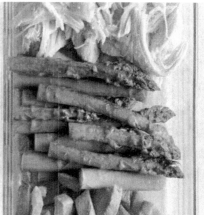

Directions

1. Preheat the oven to 425°F (218°C) and line a baking sheet with parchment paper.

2. Toss the diced sweet potato in half of the olive oil and spread across the baking sheet. Roast in the oven for 15 minutes.

3. Meanwhile, toss the asparagus in the remaining olive oil. Once the sweet potatoes have been roasting for 15 minutes, remove the pan from the oven, move the sweet potato to one side, and add the asparagus to the other side. Place back in the oven and bake for 12 to 15 more minutes, or until asparagus is tender.

4. While the veggies cook, bring a large pot of water to a boil. Drop in the chicken breasts and

poach for 15 to 20 minutes, or until cooked through. Remove the chicken from the water and shred them using two forks.

5. Divide the chicken between plates or containers and add the roasted sweet potatoes and asparagus. Top with your spices of choice.

Ingredients

3/4 Sweet Potato (medium, diced)
1 1/8 tsps Extra Virgin Olive Oil (divided)
3/4 cup Asparagus (woody ends trimmed)
5 ozs Chicken Breast (boneless, skinless)

Notes

No Asparagus
Use zucchini, green beans, broccoli, or cauliflower instead.

No Sweet Potato
Use carrots or regular potato instead.

Vegan
Swap out the chicken for roasted chickpeas or marinated lentils.

Spinach & Sausage Egg Muffins

7 ingredients · 30 minutes · 2 servings

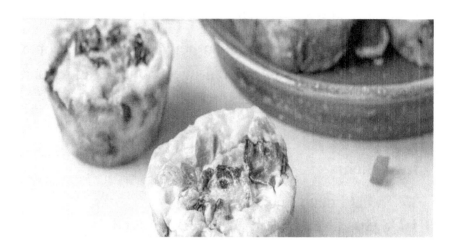

Directions

1. Preheat your oven to 350°F (176°C) and grease a muffin pan with the oil.

2. In a pan over medium-high heat, cook the sausage until no longer pink, about 5 to 8 minutes. Break it up into little pieces as it cooks. Drain the excess drippings from the pan and stir in the spinach. Cook until the spinach has wilted then remove the pan from heat to let cool slightly.

3. In a mixing bowl whisk the eggs together with the water and sea salt. Fold in the green onion.

4. Divide the sausage mixture evenly into the muffin tins and pour in the egg mixture. Bake for 15 to 18 minutes until the egg is firm to the touch

and just brown around the edges. Let the egg muffins cool slightly before removing from the pan. Enjoy!

Ingredients

1/2 tsp Extra Virgin Olive Oil
3 ozs Pork Sausage (casing removed) or ground turkey
2 cups Baby Spinach (chopped)
2 2/3 Egg
1 1/3 tbsps Water
1/16 tsp Sea Salt
1/3 stalk Green Onion (chopped)

Notes

Serving Size
One serving is two egg muffins.

More Flavor
Add chili flakes, black pepper, or hot sauce to the eggs.

Make it Vegetarian
Omit the sausage/ground turkey.

Shrimp Zoodle Stir Fry

12 ingredients · 25 minutes · 2 servings

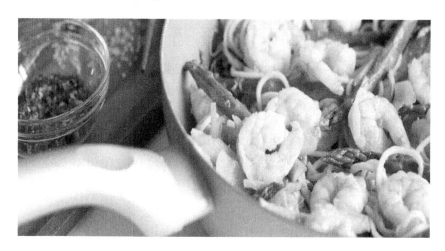

Directions

1. In a small bowl, combine the vegetable broth and tamari. Set aside.

2. Spiralize your zucchinis into noodles and set aside.

3. Place half of the coconut oil in a large frying pan and heat over medium-low heat. Add the garlic and ginger and sauté for a minute. Add the shrimp and sauté for about 3 minutes or until cooked through. (Note: Shrimp should be pink on all sides.) Transfer the shrimp to a bowl and set aside while you prepare the rest.

4. Increase heat to medium. Add remaining coconut oil to the pan along with the bell peppers, carrots, red onion, and asparagus.

Sauté for 4 minutes or until veggies are slightly tender. Add your broth/tamari mix and stir for another 4 minutes.

5. Add the shrimp back into the pan along with your zucchini noodles. Use tongs to toss and coat for 1 to 2 minutes or until zucchini noodles are slightly softened.

6. Divide stir fry onto plates and sprinkle with sesame seeds. Enjoy!

Ingredients

1/3 cup Vegetable Broth (or Chicken Broth)
1 1/3 tbsps Tamari
2 Zucchini (large)
1 1/3 tbsps Coconut Oil (divided)
2 Garlic (cloves, minced)
1 tsp Ginger (grated)
10 2/3 ozs Shrimp (peeled and deveined)
2/3 Yellow Bell Pepper (large, sliced)
2/3 cup Matchstick Carrots
2 2/3 tbsps Red Onion (diced)
2 cups Asparagus (woody ends snapped off)
2 tsps Sesame Seeds

Spicy Edamame Fried Cauliflower Rice

10 ingredients · 15 minutes · 2 servings

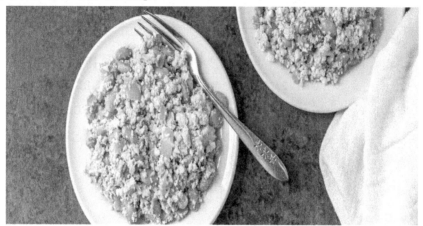

Directions

1. Heat the oil in a large pan or skillet over medium-high heat. Add the onion, bell pepper, and edamame. Cook for 3 to 5 minutes, stirring often until the onions have softened and edamame has warmed through. Add the crumbled tofu and continue to cook for about 3 minutes more until the tofu has warmed through.

2. Meanwhile, combine the tamari, garlic, ginger, and sriracha in a small mixing bowl.

3. Make a well in the middle of the pan. Pour the sauce into the well then slowly start to stir it into the tofu mixture. Continue to cook for another minute.

4. Stir in the cauliflower rice and cook until the cauliflower meets your desired texture.

Ingredients

1 1/2 tsps Sesame Oil or Extra Virgin Olive oil
1/2 Yellow Onion (finely chopped)
1 Yellow Bell Pepper (chopped)
1 1/2 cups Frozen Edamame
6 1/8 ozs Tofu (extra firm, crumbled)
3 tbsps Tamari
2 Garlic (clove, minced)
1 1/2 tsps Ginger (fresh, grated)
1 1/2 tsps Sriracha
1 cup Cauliflower Rice

Notes

Additional Toppings
Green onion, cilantro, sesame seeds, or red pepper flakes.

More Vegetables
Add carrots, peas, or baby spinach.

Zucchini Noodles with Cauliflower Alfredo

12 ingredients · 30 minutes · 2 servings

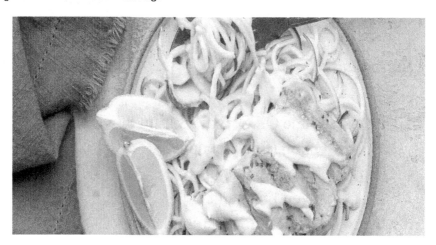

Directions

1. Bring a large pot of water to a boil under a steamer basket. Place the cauliflower florets in the steamer basket and cook for 10 to 12 minutes, or until soft.

2. In a skillet over medium heat, add half of the avocado oil and the onion. Cook for 5 to 7 minutes, until cooked through, then lower the heat to low and add the garlic. Cook for 1 to 2 minutes more. Set aside.

3. In a blender, add the steamed cauliflower, onion, garlic, nutritional yeast, coconut milk, lemon juice and 3/4 of the sea salt. Blend on high until smooth and creamy. Set aside.

4. Season the chicken breast with rosemary, garlic powder and the remaining sea salt. In a skillet over medium heat, add the remaining avocado oil. Then, add the chicken breast and cook for 8 minutes per side. Remove, let it rest for 2 to 3 minutes and then slice.

5. Plate the zucchini noodles and top with sliced chicken and cauliflower alfredo sauce. Enjoy!

Ingredients

1/4 head Cauliflower (large, chopped into florets)
1/2 tsp Avocado Oil (divided)
1/2 Yellow Onion (small, chopped)
1 Garlic (clove, minced)
2 tbsps Nutritional Yeast
1/4 cup Canned Coconut Milk
1 tbsp Lemon Juice
1/3 tsp Sea Salt (divided)
10 ozs Chicken Breast (boneless, skinless)
1 1/2 tsps Rosemary (fresh, chopped)
1/8 tsp Garlic Powder
2 Zucchini (medium, spiralized into noodles)

One Pan Steak Fajitas

9 ingredients · 20 minutes · 2 servings

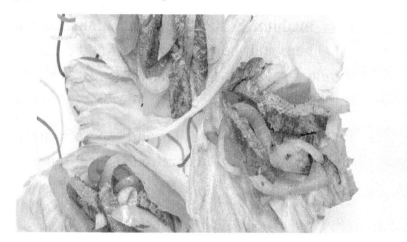

Directions

1. Preheat the oven to 400°F (205°C). Line a large baking sheet with parchment paper.

2. In a bowl, combine the chili powder, cumin, and salt. Set aside.

3. In a large mixing bowl, add your sliced peppers, onion, and steak. Drizzle with oil and then sprinkle with the seasoning. Toss until well coated. Transfer to your baking sheet and bake for 10 to 15 minutes or until the steak is cooked to your liking and the peppers are soft.

4. Scoop the steak and peppers into lettuce wraps and enjoy!

Ingredients

1 1/2 tsps Chili Powder
1/4 tsp Cumin
1/4 tsp Sea Salt
1/2 Red Bell Pepper (medium, sliced)
1/2 Orange Bell Pepper (medium, sliced)
1/2 Sweet Onion (medium, sliced)
8 ozs Flank Steak (sliced)
1 1/2 tsps Extra Virgin Olive Oil
1/2 head Iceberg Lettuce (small, leaves pulled apart)

Notes

Leftovers
Refrigerate in an airtight container for up to three days.

Serving Size
One serving is approximately three fajitas.

More Flavor
Add jalapeño peppers, paprika, and garlic powder.

Additional Toppings
Serve with avocado, lime juice, cashew cream sauce, or plain yogurt.

Seared Cod & Lemon White Beans

11 ingredients · 20 minutes · 2 servings

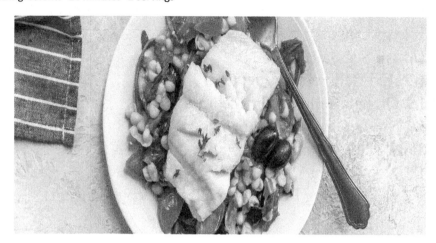

Directions

1. Season the cod with sea salt and preheat a skillet over medium heat. Add the avocado oil to the pan then add the cod. Cook for 4 minutes per side, until cooked through. Remove from the pan and set aside.

2. In the same pan, reduce the heat to medium-low and add the garlic. Cook for one minute, then add the thyme and cherry tomatoes. Cook for 2 to 3 minutes. Add the chicken broth and beans and let it simmer for 3 to 5 minutes. Add the arugula, lemon juice and olives and stir until the arugula is wilted.

3. Divide the bean and vegetable mix between plates and top with the cod. Enjoy!

Ingredients

2 Cod Fillets
1/8 tsp Sea Salt
1 tbsp Avocado Oil or Extra Virgin Olive Oil
1 Garlic (cloves, minced)
1 tsp Thyme (fresh, minced)
1/3 cup Cherry Tomatoes (halved)
1/3 cup Chicken Broth
1 cup White Navy Beans
2 1/2 cups Arugula
1 tbsp Lemon Juice
2 2/3 tbsps Pitted Kalamata Olives

Notes

Leftovers
Refrigerate in an airtight container for up to two days.

No Chicken Broth
Use vegetable broth instead.

No Arugula
Use spinach or kale instead.

Pressure Cooker Beef & Veggie Stew

11 ingredients · 1 hour · 2 servings

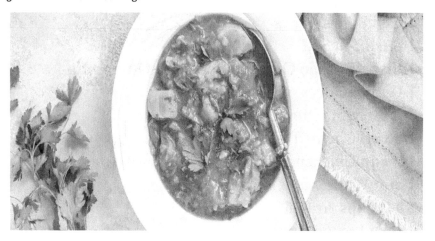

Directions

1. Turn your pressure cooker to sauté mode and add the avocado oil. Season the beef with half of the sea salt. Add it to the pressure cooker and brown on all sides, working in batches if necessary.

2. Turn off the sauté mode and add all other ingredients, including the remaining salt. Stir to combine. Put the lid on the pressure cooker and change to meat/stew mode. Cook for 35 minutes and then do a quick release. Serve and enjoy!

Ingredients

1/2 tsp Avocado Oil
8 ozs Stewing Beef (diced into cubes)
8 fl ozs Bone Broth

1/4 tsp Sea Salt (divided)
1/4 cup Pureed Pumpkin
1 1/2 tsps Apple Cider Vinegar
1 Garlic (clove, minced)
1 Parsnip (peeled, chopped)
2 1/2 White Button Mushrooms (halved)
1/2 Yellow Onion (medium, sliced in large chunks)
1/2 tsp Thyme (dried)

Notes

Serving Size
One serving is approximately 2 cups.

Want it Thicker
After cooking, create a slurry by mixing 1 tbsp arrowroot powder with a little water and add to the stew. Repeat as needed for desired thickness.

No Pumpkin
Use butternut squash purée instead.

Crunchy Veggies
Vegetables can turn soft in the pressure cooker. If you prefer crunchy veggies, steam them on the stove separately, then add them to the meal when it's done.

Week Five

Week Five: no sugar, low glycemic, no dairy, corn free, gluten free, low lectin, soy free. Limit one caffeinated drink each morning. Drink water, spearmint tea, green tea.

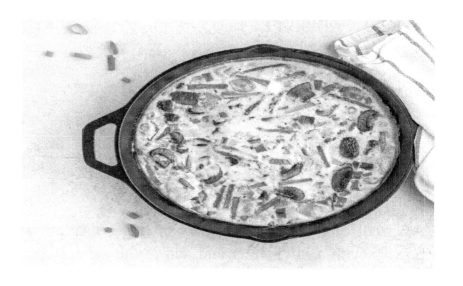

Week Five Meal Plan

	Mon	Tue	Wed	Thu	Fri	Sat	Sun
Breakfast	Oil-Free Scrambled Egg Whites	Fruit & Egg Snack Plate	Turkey Sausage Scramble	Eggs n' Guac Breakfast Bowl	Fried Egg	Triple Berry Protein Bowl	Asparagus & Mushroom Frittata
	Sweet Potato Hashbrowns	Grain-Free Flax Bread		Blueberries	Grain-Free Flax Bread		
Lunch	One Pot Poached Chicken with Broccoli & Sweet Potato	Sheet Pan Roasted Chicken & Veggies	Simple Salmon Salad	Brussels Sprouts Slaw with Chicken	Turkey & Vegetable Soup	One Pan Lemon Garlic Shrimp, Broccoli & Cauliflower Rice	Balsamic Dijon Chicken Thighs with Broccoli
	Broccoli & Mushroom Fried Rice				Coconut Chive Flatbread		
Snack 2	Fresh Strawberries	Carrot Sticks	Fresh Strawberries	Tuna & Kale Chips	Brazil Nuts & Blueberries	Green Lemonade	Green Lemonade
	Salmon Salad Lettuce Wraps		Brazil Nuts		Carrot Sticks	Hard Boiled Eggs	Blackberries & Pistachios
Dinner	Sheet Pan Roasted Chicken & Veggies	Mayo-Dijon Salmon with Broccoli	Brussels Sprouts Slaw with Chicken	Turkey & Vegetable Soup	One Pan Lemon Garlic Shrimp, Broccoli & Cauliflower	Balsamic Dijon Chicken Thighs with Broccoli	Slow Cooker Cod & Sea Veggie Soup
					Steamed Asparagus		

Oil-Free Scrambled Egg Whites

1 ingredient · 10 minutes · 3 servings

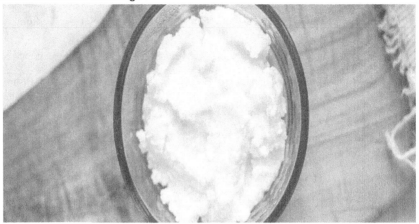

Directions

1. Add the egg whites to a cold saucepan. Place over low to low-medium heat and stir continuously with a heat-safe spatula until fluffy and cooked through, about 10 minutes.

2. Transfer to a plate and enjoy!

Ingredients

3 cups Egg Whites

Notes

Leftovers
Refrigerate in an airtight container for up to three days.

Additional Toppings
Black pepper, crushed red pepper flakes, herbs, or salsa.

Sweet Potato Hashbrowns

4 ingredients · 20 minutes · 3 servings

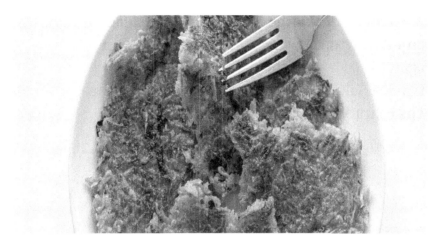

Directions

1. Using your hands and a paper towel or kitchen towel, squeeze as much liquid out of the shredded sweet potato as possible.

2. In a mixing bowl, combine the sweet potato, arrowroot powder and salt.

3. Heat oil in a cast iron skillet over medium heat. Sprinkle the sweet potato evenly across the skillet to form a thin layer. Press down with a spatula and cook on each side for 4 to 5 minutes, or until brown and crispy.

4. Transfer to a towel-lined plate to absorb any excess oil. Let cool slightly and enjoy!

Ingredients

1 1/2 Sweet Potato (large, peeled, and shredded)
1/4 cup Arrowroot Powder (this is substitute for cornstarch)
1/3 tsp Sea Salt
3 tbsps Extra Virgin Olive Oil

Notes

Leftovers
Refrigerate in an airtight container for up to five days.

More Flavor
Add garlic and/or onion powder to the sweet potato mixture.

Additional Toppings
Top with avocado, spinach, sausage patty or poached egg.

Fruit & Egg Snack Plate

3 ingredients · 20 minutes · 1 serving

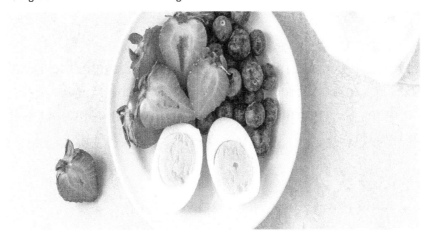

Directions

1. Place eggs in a saucepan and cover with water. Bring to a boil over high heat then turn off the heat but keep the saucepan on the hot burner. Cover and let sit for 10 to 12 minutes. Transfer the eggs to a bowl of cold water and let the eggs sit until cool enough to handle.

2. Peel and slice the hard boiled egg and serve with the blueberries and strawberries. Enjoy!

Ingredients

1 Egg
1/2 cup Blueberries
1/2 cup Strawberries (halved)

Notes

Leftovers
Store the eggs and fruit separately. Refrigerate the hard boiled eggs in a covered container with the shell on for up to seven days. Refrigerate the fruit in an airtight container for up to two days.

Serving Size
One serving is one egg and one cup of fruit.

Turkey Sausage Scramble

4 ingredients · 10 minutes · 1 serving

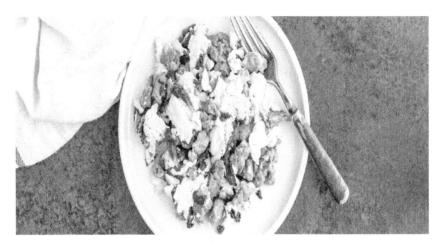

Directions

1. Heat a pan over medium heat then add the sausage to the pan. Brown for five to six minutes or until cooked through, breaking it up as it cooks. Add the spinach to the pan and move it around until it's wilted.

2. Move the sausage and spinach to one side of the pan and pour the eggs into the empty side. Stir the eggs frequently as they cook and incorporate the spinach and sausage into the egg once the eggs are cooked through. Season with salt and pepper if needed and enjoy!

Ingredients

4 1/16 ozs Turkey Sausage (casing removed)
1 cup Baby Spinach (chopped)
2 Eggs (whisked)
Sea Salt & Black Pepper (to taste)

Notes

Leftovers
Best enjoyed immediately. Sausage can be cooked ahead of time and reheated in the pan to save time.

More Flavor
Add onion, mushrooms, or bell pepper.

Additional Toppings
Hot sauce, avocado, or sugar free salsa.

No Spinach
Use kale instead.

No Turkey Sausage
Use pork, chicken, or beef sausage instead. Use crumbled tofu to make it vegetarian.

Eggs n' Guac Breakfast Bowl

7 ingredients · 15 minutes · 1 serving

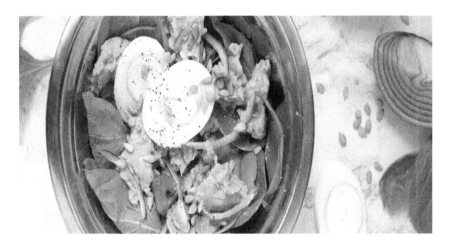

Directions

1. Place eggs in a pot of cold water, bring to a boil, then simmer for 5-6 minutes. Peel the eggs and slice in half.

2. Make guacamole by mashing avocado and mixing with lemon, sea salt and pepper to taste.

3. Divide spinach into bowls and top with guacamole, egg, red onion, and olive oil. Enjoy!

Ingredients

2 Egg
1/2 Avocado
1/4 Lemon (juiced)

Sea Salt & Black Pepper (to taste)
2 cups Baby Spinach
1 tbsp Red Onion (thinly sliced)
1 1/2 tsps Extra Virgin Olive Oil

Notes

Storage
Keep refrigerated in an air-tight container up to 3 days.

Prep Ahead
Hard boil your eggs in advance to save time.

Make it Spicy
Add chili flakes.

Make it Vegan
Skip the eggs and add cooked chickpeas instead.

Extra Toppings
Try adding hot sauce, sunflower seeds, pumpkin seeds, or hemp hearts.

Triple Berry Protein Bowl

7 ingredients · 10 minutes · 1 serving

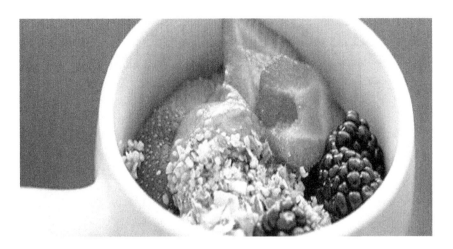

Directions

1. Wash berries and place in bowl(s). Sprinkle berries with hemp seeds and slivered almonds. Top with almond butter and pour almond milk over top. Enjoy!

Ingredients

1/2 cup Strawberries (sliced)
1/2 cup Blueberries
1/2 cup Blackberries
1 tbsp Almond Butter
1 tbsp Hemp Seeds
2 tbsps Slivered Almonds
1/4 cup Unsweetened Almond Milk

Asparagus & Mushroom Frittata

7 ingredients · 25 minutes · 1 serving

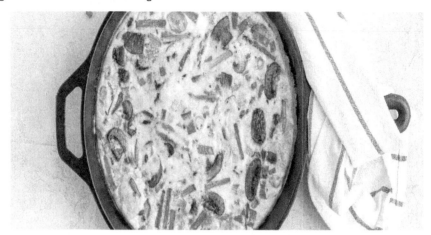

Directions

1. Preheat the oven to 400°F (204°C).
2. Add the eggs and water to a bowl and whisk well. Set aside.
3. Heat the oil in a cast-iron skillet, or another oven-proof skillet, over medium heat. Add the mushrooms and asparagus and cook until the mushrooms have softened, and the asparagus is fork-tender, five to seven minutes. Stir in the green onion, salt, and pepper, and continue to cook for another minute until the green onions have softened.
4. Pour the whisked eggs into the skillet with the vegetables and let the eggs cook for about 30 seconds or until they just begin to set, before gently stirring with a spatula to ensure the

vegetables are well incorporated into the eggs. Transfer the skillet to the oven.

5. Bake for 12 to 15 minutes or until eggs have set and are firm to the touch in the center of the pan. Let sit for five minutes before cutting into wedges. Season with additional salt and pepper if needed and enjoy!

Ingredients

2 Egg
1 tbsp Water
3/4 tsp Extra Virgin Olive Oil
1/2 cup Mushrooms (sliced)
1/4 cup Asparagus (sliced)
1/2 stalk Green Onion (chopped)
Sea Salt & Black Pepper (to taste)

Notes

Serving Size
A 10-inch cast-iron pan was used for four servings.

More Flavor
Add fresh or dried herbs, garlic, or red pepper flakes.

One Pot Poached Chicken with Broccoli & Sweet Potato

6 ingredients · 20 minutes · 1 serving

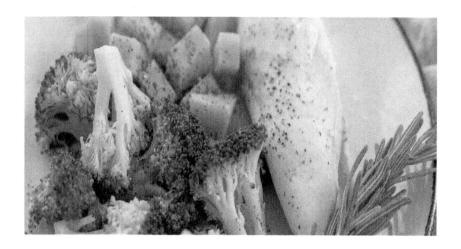

Directions

1. In a pot over medium-high heat, add chicken followed by the remaining ingredients. Bring to a boil, reduce heat to a simmer and close the pan. Let simmer until chicken is cooked through, about 15-20 minutes.

2. Using a slotted spoon, scoop out the chicken and veggies. Shred the chicken, season with sea salt and black pepper, and drizzle with broth. Save the leftover broth for future use. Enjoy!

Ingredients

5 ozs Chicken Breast (skinless, boneless)
1 1/2 tsps Apple Cider Vinegar
1 cup Water
1/2 Sweet Potato (medium, diced)
1 cup Broccoli (chopped into florets)
Sea Salt & Black Pepper (to taste)

Notes

More Flavour
Use low sodium chicken or vegetable broth instead of water, add herbs, garlic cloves and/or onion wedges.

No Broccoli or Sweet Potato
Use carrots, celery, or cauliflower instead.

Leftovers
Refrigerate chicken in an air-tight container up to 3 days, and the broth up to 2 days, or freeze for up to 2 months.

Broccoli & Mushroom Fried Rice

10 ingredients · 15 minutes · 1 serving

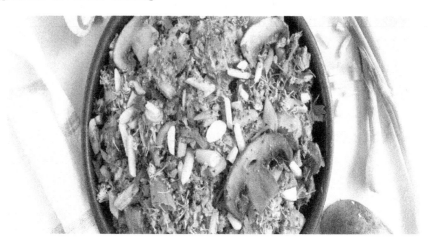

Directions

1. Add the broccoli florets to a food processor and pulse until a rice consistency forms.

2. Heat a large pan over medium heat and add in the avocado oil. Once the oil is warmed, add in the broccoli, mushrooms, and garlic. Cook for 10 minutes.

3. Once the ingredients are cooked through, add in the coconut aminos, almonds, onion powder and sea salt. Cook for roughly 3 minutes, stirring often to combine the flavors. Remove from heat.

4. Top with green onions and cilantro.

Ingredients

1/2 cup Broccoli (chopped into small florets)
3/4 tsp Avocado Oil
1/2 cup Mushrooms (sliced)
1/8 Garlic (clove, minced)
3/4 tsp Coconut aminos (substitute for low sodium soy sauce)
1 tbsp Almonds (slivered)
3/4 tsp Onion Powder
1/4 tsp Sea Salt
3/4 stalk Green Onion (chopped)
1 tbsp Cilantro (chopped)

Notes

Leftovers
Refrigerate in an airtight container for up to three days. For best results, reheat in a skillet.

Nut-Free
Omit the almonds or use sunflower or sesame seeds instead.

More Protein
Top with a fried egg or stir in a scrambled egg.

Coconut Chive Flatbread

7 ingredients · 15 minutes · 1 serving

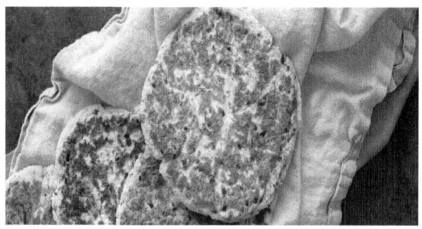

Directions

1. In a mixing bowl, combine the flour, psyllium husk, dried chives, baking soda and salt.

2. Add the oil and water. Knead with your hands and form a ball. The texture should be soft and elastic, but not sticky. If the dough is too wet, add more psyllium husk. If it is too dry, add water.

3. Cut the dough into the according number of recipe servings. Roll into balls.

4. Place one dough ball between two sheets of parchment paper and use a rolling pin to roll it out evenly to approximately 8 inches wide. Repeat until the remaining balls of dough are shaped.

5. Very lightly grease a cast iron or non-stick pan and place over medium-high heat. Cook for 2 to 3 minutes. Flip and cook for another 1 to 2 minutes. Grease the pan as needed and repeat until all servings are cooked. Enjoy!

Ingredients

2 tbsps Coconut Flour
1 1/2 tsps Psyllium Husk Powder
1 tbsp Dried Chives
1/16 tsp Baking Soda
1/8 tsp Sea Salt
3/4 tsp Extra Virgin Olive Oil (plus extra for greasing)
1/4 cup Water (warm)

Notes

Leftovers
Stack between layers of parchment paper and refrigerate in an airtight container or storage bag for up to five days. Freeze for up to one month. Reheat on a pan or in the oven for best results.

Serving Size
One serving is equal to one 8-inch flatbread.

Salmon Salad Lettuce Wraps

6 ingredients · 5 minutes · 3 servings

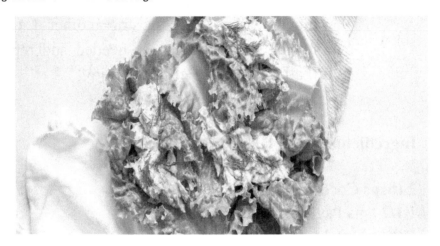

Directions

1. In a bowl, combine the salmon, coconut yogurt, dill, lemon juice and salt. Adjust flavours as desired.

2. Scoop the mixture onto the lettuce leaves and enjoy!

Ingredients

15 ozs Canned Wild Salmon (drained)
1 cup Unsweetened Coconut Yogurt
1/4 cup Fresh Dill (minced)
1 tbsp Lemon Juice
1/2 tsp Sea Salt
1/2 head Green Lettuce (separated into leaves and washed)

Notes

Leftovers
Refrigerate the salmon mixture and lettuce leaves in separate airtight containers for up to three days.

Serving Size
One serving equals approximately three salmon stuffed lettuce leaves.

Additional Toppings
Add cucumber, celery, red onion, or tomato.

No Coconut Yogurt
Use Greek yogurt.

Tuna & Kale Chips

4 ingredients · 10 minutes · 1 serving

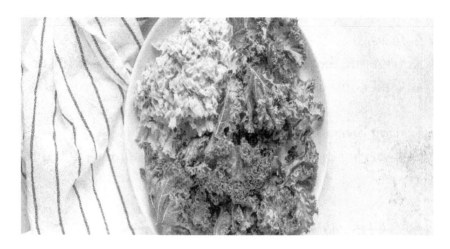

Directions

1. Preheat the oven to 350°F (175°C). Line a baking sheet with parchment paper.

2. Arrange the kale across the baking sheet. Bake in the oven for 10 to 15 minutes or until crispy (watch closely for burning).

3. Meanwhile, mix the tuna, coconut yogurt, and salt together in a bowl. Serve with the kale chips and enjoy!

Ingredients

2 cups Kale Leaves (tough stems removed, torn into pieces)
1/2 can Tuna in water (drained)
2 tbsps Unsweetened Coconut Yogurt
1/8 tsp Sea Salt (to taste)

Notes

Leftovers
Refrigerate in an airtight container for up to three days.

Additional Toppings
Add chopped celery and red onion to the tuna.

No Tuna
Use canned salmon instead.

Sheet Pan Roasted Chicken & Veggies

9 ingredients · 30 minutes · 2 servings

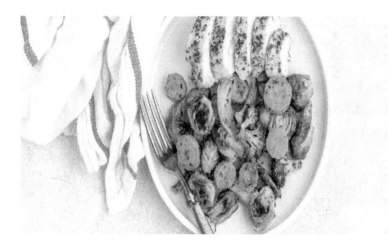

Directions

1. Preheat the oven to 400°F (204°C) and line a baking sheet with parchment paper.

2. Add the veggies and the chicken to the baking sheeting then drizzle with the oil and season with the Italian seasoning, garlic powder, and salt.

3. Bake for 25 minutes or until the chicken is cooked through and the veggies are tender. Season with additional salt if needed. Divide between plates and enjoy!

Ingredients

2 cups Brussels Sprouts (halved or quartered)
1 cup Broccoli (cut into small florets)
1 Carrot (peeled, thinly sliced)
1 Yellow Onion (medium, cut into wedges)
8 ozs Chicken Breast
1 tbsp Extra Virgin Olive Oil
1 tsp Italian Seasoning
1/2 tsp Garlic Powder
1/4 tsp Sea Salt

Notes

Leftovers
Refrigerate in an airtight container for up to three days.

More Flavor
Add other dried herbs and spices.

No Chicken Breast
Use chicken thighs or drumsticks instead.

Serve it With
Cauliflower rice, quinoa, brown rice, roasted potatoes, or mashed sweet potato.

Mayo-Dijon Salmon with Broccoli

6 ingredients · 15 minutes · 2 servings

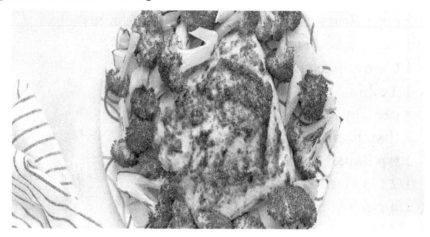

Directions

1. Preheat the oven to 450°F (230°C) and line a baking sheet with parchment paper.

2. In a bowl, mix together the mayonnaise and Dijon mustard.

3. Place the salmon fillets on the baking sheet and season with salt and pepper. Coat the salmon generously in the mayo-Dijon mixture.

4. Toss the broccoli florets in the oil and season with salt and pepper. Add them to the baking sheet, arranging them around the salmon fillets.

5. Bake the salmon and broccoli in the oven for 10

to 15 minutes, or until the salmon flakes with a fork and is browned on top. Divide onto plates and enjoy!

Ingredients

2 tbsps Mayonnaise
1 tbsp Dijon Mustard
12 ozs Salmon Fillet
Sea Salt & Black Pepper (to taste)
5 cups Broccoli (sliced into small florets)
1 tbsp Extra Virgin Olive Oil

Notes

Leftovers
Refrigerate in an airtight container for up to two days.

Serving Size
One serving equals approximately six ounces of salmon and 2 1/2 cups of broccoli.

Turkey & Vegetable Soup

11 ingredients · 50 minutes · 2 servings

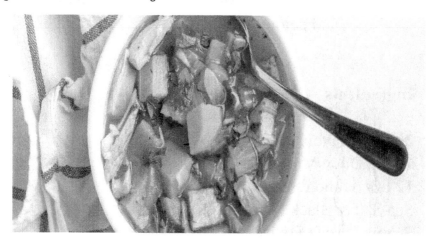

Directions

1. Heat the oil in a large pot over medium heat.

2. Add the onion and cook until it begins to soften, about 5 minutes. Add in the garlic, thyme and salt and continue cooking for one minute more.

3. Add the sweet potato, carrots, celery, and turkey. Stir to combine then add the chicken broth to the pot along with the parsley.

4. Bring soup to a gentle boil then reduce the heat to low and cover with a lid. Simmer for 40 to 45 minutes or until the vegetables are very tender. Season with additional salt if needed. Serve and enjoy!

Ingredients

1 tsp Extra Virgin Olive Oil
1/3 Yellow Onion (chopped)
1 Garlic (clove, minced)
1/3 tsp Dried Thyme
1/3 tsp Sea Salt
1/3 Sweet Potato (peeled, cut into 1/2-inch cubes)
1/3 Carrot (peeled, chopped)
2/3 stalk Celery (chopped)
3 1/2 ozs Turkey or Chicken Breast, Cooked (roughly chopped)
2 cups Chicken Broth
1/3 cup Parsley (chopped)

Notes

Serving Size
One serving is approximately 1 1/2 cups of soup.

Additional Toppings
Serve the soup over top of cooked brown rice or cooked spaghetti squash.

One Pan Lemon Garlic Shrimp, Broccoli & Cauliflower Rice

8 ingredients · 30 minutes · 2 servings

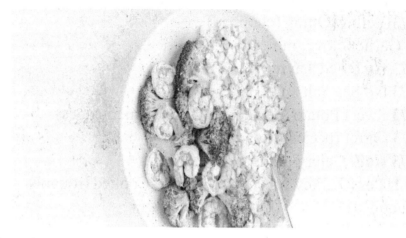

Directions

1. Preheat the oven to 400°F (205°C) and line a baking sheet with parchment paper.

2. Place the cauliflower rice on one side of the baking sheet and the broccoli florets in the middle, leaving room for the shrimp. Drizzle with half of the oil and half of the salt. Toss to coat.

3. Place in the oven and bake for 15 minutes, turning broccoli halfway through.

4. Meanwhile, in a small bowl, add the remaining oil, salt, lemon juice, smashed garlic cloves, and black pepper. Whisk well and set aside.

5. Remove the baking sheet from the oven and add the shrimp. Pour half of the lemon garlic dressing on top of the shrimp and broccoli. Discard the smashed garlic cloves. Place back in the oven for seven to eight minutes or until the shrimp is cooked.

6. To serve, divide the cauliflower rice, broccoli, and shrimp into bowls. Top with remaining lemon garlic dressing. Enjoy!

Ingredients

3 cups Cauliflower Rice
3 cups Broccoli (florets)
1 tbsp Extra Virgin Olive Oil (divided)
3/4 tsp Sea Salt (divided)
1 Lemon (juiced)
2 Garlic (cloves, smashed)
1/4 tsp Black Pepper
8 ozs Shrimp (peeled, deveined, tails removed).

Steamed Asparagus

1 ingredient · 10 minutes · 1 serving

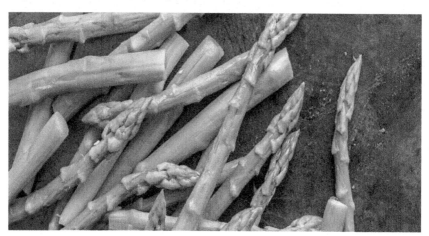

Directions

1. Set the asparagus in a steaming basket over boiling water and cover. Steam for 3 to 5 minutes for thin asparagus, or 6 to 8 minutes for thick asparagus. Enjoy!

Ingredients

1 cup Asparagus (woody ends trimmed, chopped in half)

Notes

Leftovers
Refrigerate in an airtight container up to 5 days.

Serving Size
One serving is equal to approximately one cup of cooked asparagus.

Balsamic Dijon Chicken Thighs with Broccoli

9 ingredients · 30 minutes · 2 servings

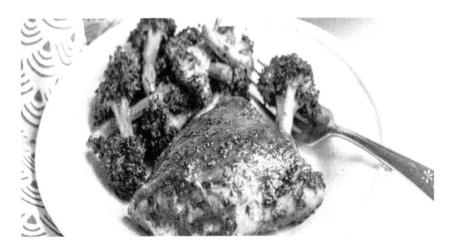

Directions

1. Preheat oven to 400°F (204°C) and line a baking sheet with parchment paper.

2. Place chicken in the center of the baking sheet and arrange the broccoli in a single layer around the chicken. Drizzle oil over chicken and veggies then add half of the salt, pepper, and garlic powder. Using your hands, toss or rub the spices evenly all over the chicken and the broccoli. Bake in the oven for 15 minutes.

3. Meanwhile, whisk the Dijon mustard, balsamic vinegar, oregano, and remaining salt together. Set aside.

4. After the chicken has baked for 15 minutes,

remove from oven and brush half the Dijon mixture on top of the chicken and lightly over the broccoli. Return to oven and bake for 10 more minutes.

5. After 10 minutes, repeat step 4 with remaining Dijon mixture. Place back into the oven and continue to bake for 5 to 10 more minutes, or until chicken is cooked through and broccoli is very tender.

6. Remove from oven and serve immediately.

Ingredients

8 ozs Chicken Thighs (skinless, boneless)
3 cups Broccoli (chopped into florets)
1 tbsp Extra Virgin Olive Oil
1/2 tsp Sea Salt (divided)
1/2 tsp Black Pepper
1/2 tsp Garlic Powder
1 tbsp Dijon Mustard
1/4 cup Balsamic Vinegar
1 tsp Oregano (dried)

Week Six

Week Six: sugar free, low glycemic, heart healthy, immune boosting, gluten free. Protein powders can be omitted from any recipe.

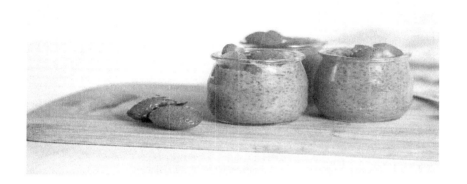

Week Six Meal Plan

	Mon	Tue	Wed	Thu	Fri	Sat	Sun
Breakfast	Creamy Blueberry Smoothie	Chia Oats with Kiwi	Creamy Blueberry Smoothie	Chia Oats with Kiwi	Avocado Breakfast Toast	Cinnamon Oatmeal Pancakes Fried Egg	Chocolate Strawberry Chia Pudding
Lunch	Creamy Carrot Soup Grain-Free Flax Bread	One Pan Chicken Fajita Bowls	Zucchini Noodle Lasagna	Citrus Glazed Salmon House Salad	Grilled Mediterranean Chicken Kabobs	Turkey Chili	Cobb Salad
Snack 2	Smoked Salmon Wrapped Avocado	Carrot Sticks	Smoked Salmon Wrapped Avocado	Hummus & Veggies Snack Box	Apples & Almonds	Blackberries	Plum
Dinner	One Pan Chicken Fajita Bowls Wild Rice	Zucchini Noodle Lasagna	Citrus Glazed Salmon	Grilled Mediterranean Chicken Kabobs	Turkey Chili	Ginger Chicken Bowl	Spiced Cauliflower Rice Bowl

Creamy Blueberry Smoothie

7 ingredients · 5 minutes · 1 serving

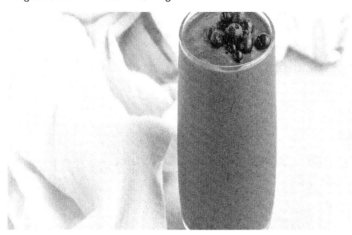

Directions

1. Add all ingredients to a blender and blend until smooth. Pour into a glass and enjoy!

Ingredients

1 cup Frozen Blueberries

1 cup Frozen Cauliflower

1/2 cup Unsweetened Coconut Yogurt

1/4 cup Vanilla Protein Powder

1 tbsp Chia Seeds

1 Lemon (small, juiced)

1 cup Water

Notes

Additional Toppings
Add spinach, avocado, kale, or other berries (without seeds) to your smoothie.

Extra Creamy
Use almond milk or oat milk instead of water.

Lemon
One lemon yields approximately 1/4 cup of lemon juice.

Protein Powder
This recipe was developed and tested using a plant-based protein powder. If using another type of protein powder, note that results may vary. Omit protein powder if desired.

Chia Oats with Kiwi

4 ingredients · 10 minutes · 2 servings

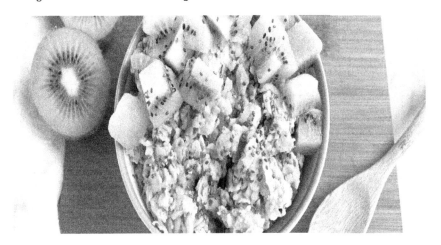

Directions

1. In a small saucepan, bring the water to a boil and add the oats and chia seeds. Reduce to a simmer and cook for 4 to 5 minutes or until cooked through. Be sure to stir often.

2. Divide the oatmeal between bowls and top with kiwi. Enjoy!

Ingredients

1 cup Water
1 cup Oats (rolled)
2 tbsps Chia Seeds
1 Kiwi (chopped)

Notes

Leftovers
Refrigerate in an airtight container for up to four days. For best results, reheat with additional liquid over the stove or in the microwave.

Serving Size
One serving is equal to half a cup of oatmeal and half of a kiwi.

More Flavor
Add cinnamon

Additional Toppings
Add nuts, seeds, and berries.

Avocado Breakfast Toast

5 ingredients · 25 minutes · 2 servings

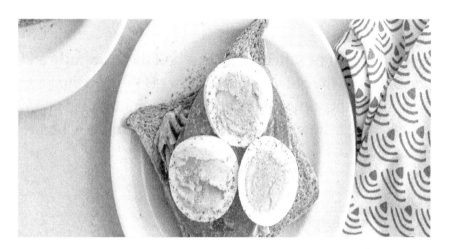

Directions

1. Spread the mashed avocado on the toast then arrange the tomato and hard-boiled egg slices on top. Season with salt and pepper to taste and enjoy!

Ingredients

1 Avocado (small, mashed)
2 slices Whole Grain Bread (toasted)
1 Tomato (small, sliced)
2 Egg (hard-boiled, peeled and sliced)
Sea Salt & Black Pepper (to taste)

Notes

How to Hard-Boil Eggs
Bring a small pot of salted water to a boil then carefully add the eggs. Cover the pot with a lid. Turn off the heat but keep the pot on the hot burner. Let stand for 12 minutes then drain. Place eggs in a bowl of ice water for 10 minutes before peeling.

Gluten-Free
Use gluten-free bread.

No Hard-Boiled Eggs
Use fried, scrambled, or poached eggs instead.

Likes it Spicy
Add a pinch of chili flakes or hot sauce to the mashed avocado.

Cinnamon Oatmeal Pancakes

9 ingredients · 25 minutes · 1 serving

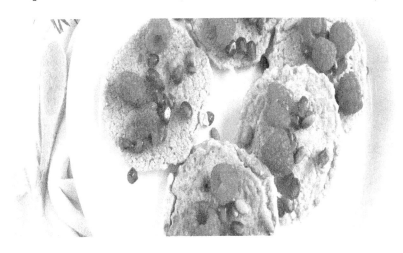

Directions

1. In a food processor, process the rolled oats until it creates a flour-like consistency. Add the baking powder and cinnamon and pulse to combine.

2. Add the egg, almond milk, and half of the coconut oil to the oat mixture and process until well combined.

3. Add the remaining coconut oil to a large skillet and place over medium heat. Once hot, pour the batter into skillet the to form one pancake about 3-inches wide.

4. Once small holes begin to appear in the surface of

the pancake, flip over. Cook each side approximately 3 to 4 minutes. Repeat until the batter is finished.

5. Top the pancakes with pomegranate seeds, raspberries, and pumpkin seeds. Enjoy!

Ingredients

2/3 cup Oats (rolled)
1/4 tsp Baking Powder
2/3 tsp Cinnamon
1/4 Egg
1/3 cup Unsweetened Almond Milk
1/4 tsps Coconut Oil (divided)
2 1/3 tsps Pomegranate Seeds
1 1/16 tbsps Raspberries
1/3 tsps Pumpkin Seeds

Notes

Serving Size
One serving is roughly 2 pancakes.

Additional Toppings
Add nuts, seeds, or berries on top.

Fried Egg

1 ingredients · 5 minutes · 1 serving

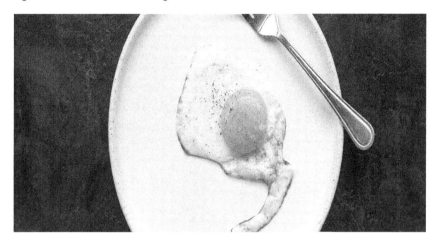

Directions

1. In a medium pan, heat the olive oil over medium heat.

2. Crack the egg in the pan and cook until the whites are set, and the yolk is cooked to your liking. Transfer to a plate and enjoy!

Ingredients

1/4 tsp Extra Virgin Olive oil
1 Egg
Sea Salt & Black Pepper (to taste)

Notes

No Olive Oil
Use unsalted butter but not margarine.

Chocolate Strawberry Chia Pudding

4 ingredients · 30 minutes · 1 serving

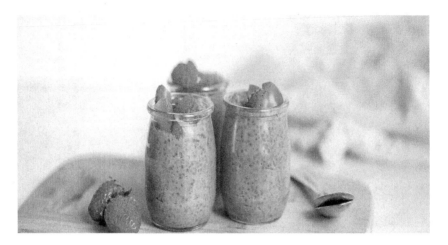

Directions

1. In a large bowl, combine the chia seeds with the coconut milk and the protein powder. Whisk well, making sure all the seeds are incorporated. Refrigerate for at least 20 minutes or overnight to thicken.

2. Top the chia pudding with the strawberries and enjoy!

Ingredients

2 tbsps Chia Seeds
1/2 cup Plain Coconut Milk (unsweetened, from the carton)
2 tbsps Chocolate Protein Powder
1/2 cup Strawberries (halved)

Notes

Leftovers
Refrigerate in an airtight container for up to four days.

No Protein Powder
Use raw cacao powder or cocoa powder instead of protein powder, using half the amount.

Protein Powder
This recipe was developed and tested using a plant-based protein powder.

Creamy Carrot Soup

11 ingredients · 50 minutes · 1 serving

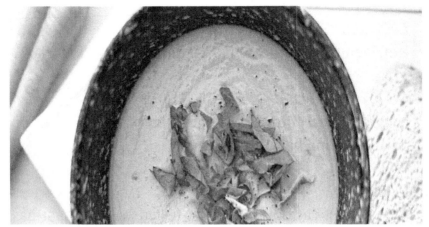

Directions

1. In a large pot, heat olive oil over medium heat. Stir in onion, garlic, carrots, cumin, and turmeric. Season with salt and pepper to taste. Sautee for about 10 minutes or until veggies start to brown.

2. Add in vegetable broth. Cover with lid and let simmer for 30 minutes.

3. After 30 minutes, pour in almond milk and stir well. Transfer soup to a blender to puree. Always be careful to leave a hole for the steam to escape or the lid will pop off while blending. Blend in batches and transfer back to pot. Taste and season with more sea salt and pepper if desired.

4. Ladle soup into bowls. Garnish with chopped

spinach and drizzle with a squeeze of lemon wedge. Serve with a slice of bread for dipping and/or a mixed greens salad.

Ingredients

3/4 tsp Extra Virgin Olive Oil
Carrot (chopped into 1 inch rounds)
1/4 Sweet Onion (chopped)
1/2 Garlic (cloves, minced)
1/4 tsp Cumin
1/4 tsp Turmeric
Sea Salt & Black Pepper (to taste)
3/4 cup Vegetable Broth
1/4 cup Unsweetened Almond Milk
1/4 Lemon (cut into wedges)
1/4 cup Baby Spinach (chopped)

Notes

Leftovers
Refrigerate in an airtight container for up to four days. Freeze for up to three months.

Serving Size
One serving is roughly 1 1/2 to 2 cups of soup.

Cobb Salad

9 ingredients · 25 minutes · 1 serving

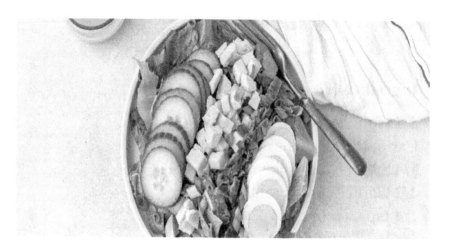

Directions

1. Place the eggs in a saucepan and cover with water. Bring to a boil over high heat then turn off the heat but keep the saucepan on the hot burner. Cover and let sit for 10 to 12 minutes. Transfer the eggs to a bowl of cold water and let the eggs sit until cool enough to handle. Peel and slice.

2. Meanwhile, cook the bacon in a large pan over medium heat for about five minutes per side or until the bacon is cooked through and crispy. Transfer to a paper towel-lined plate to let the bacon cool slightly then chop into small pieces.

3. To a jar add the oil, lemon juice, and mustard. Shake to combine.

4. To serve, divide the romaine between plates

and top with the chicken, egg, bacon, cucumber, and green onion. Drizzle the dressing on top. Enjoy!

Ingredients

1 Egg
1 slice Bacon (cut off excess fat)
1 tbsp Extra Virgin Olive Oil
1 tbsp Lemon Juice
1/4 tsp Dijon Mustard
4 leaves Romaine (chopped) or spinach
3 1/2 ozs Chicken Breast, Cooked (chopped)
1/4 Cucumber (sliced)
1 stalk Green Onion (chopped, greens parts only)

Notes

Leftovers
Refrigerate in an airtight container for up to three days.

More Flavor
Add dried herbs, fresh garlic, salt, and/or pepper to the dressing.

Smoked Salmon Wrapped Avocado

2 ingredients · 5 minutes · 2 servings

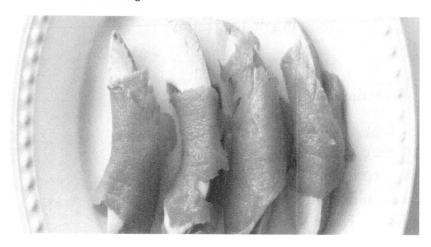

Directions

1. Slice the avocado and wrap each slice with the smoked salmon. Transfer to a plate and enjoy!

Ingredients

1 Avocado

3 1/2 ozs Smoked Salmon (sliced).

Notes

Leftovers
Refrigerate in an airtight container for up to two days.

Easier handling
Wrap the salmon around smaller pieces and pin with a toothpick

Hummus & Veggies Snack Box

4 ingredients · 5 minutes · 1 serving

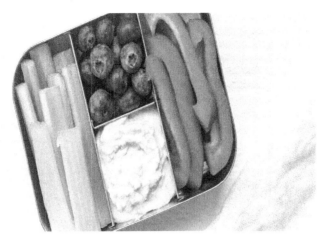

Directions

1. Assemble all ingredients into a storage container and refrigerate until ready to eat. Enjoy!

Ingredients

1/2 Red Bell Pepper (sliced)
2 stalks Celery (cut into small stalks)
1/3 cup Blueberries
1/4 cup Hummus

Notes

Storage
Refrigerate in an airtight container up to 2 days.

No Hummus
Use guacamole instead.

One Pan Chicken Fajita Bowls

8 ingredients · 40 minutes · 2 servings

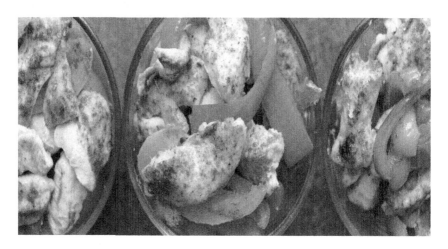

Directions

1. Preheat oven to 375°F (191°C) and line a baking sheet with parchment paper.

2. In a large bowl, toss the sliced bell peppers with the olive oil. Transfer to a baking sheet and add the sliced chicken breast. Sprinkle with cumin, chilli powder, salt and pepper.

3. Bake for 30 minutes, or until chicken is cooked through.

4. Divide between bowls or containers. Enjoy!

Ingredients

1 Red Bell Pepper (sliced)
1/2 Orange Bell Pepper (sliced)
1/2 Green Bell Pepper (sliced)
1 tbsp Extra Virgin Olive Oil
8 ozs Chicken Breast
1 1/2 tsps Cumin
1 1/2 tsps Chili Powder
Sea Salt & Black Pepper (to taste)

Notes

Leftovers
Keeps well in the fridge for 3 days.

More Carbs
Serve with brown rice, quinoa, or black beans.

Vegan/Vegetarian
Use tofu or chickpeas instead of chicken.

Wild Rice

3 ingredients · 45 minutes · 2 servings

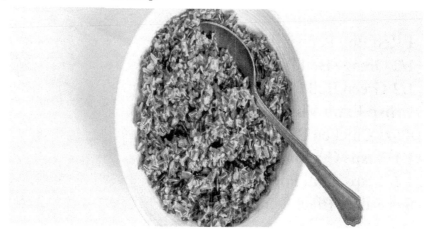

Directions

1. Combine the wild rice, water, and salt together in a saucepan. Place over high heat and bring to a boil. Once boiling, reduce heat to a simmer and cover with a lid. Let simmer for 40 minutes or until the water is absorbed. Remove lid and fluff with a fork. Enjoy!

Ingredients

1/2 cup Wild Rice
1 1/2 cups Water
1/4 tsp Sea Salt

Notes

Leftovers
Refrigerate in an airtight container for up to five days.

Serving Size
One serving is about 1/2 cup cooked wild rice.

More Flavor
Use chicken or vegetable broth instead of water.

Zucchini Noodle Lasagna

9 ingredients · 20 minutes · 2 servings

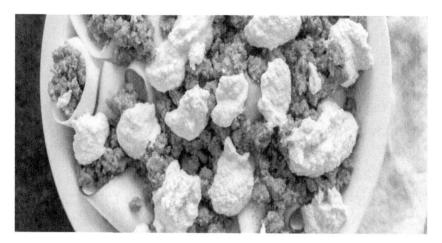

Directions

1. Heat oil in a saucepan over medium-high heat. Cook the ground beef for about 5 minutes and drain any excess liquid. Season with half the salt and add the tomato sauce. Let simmer for about 10 minutes.

2. Meanwhile, add the soaked cashews, lemon juice, nutritional yeast, water, and remaining salt to a blender. Blend until creamy.

3. Slice your zucchini lengthwise using a peeler. Divide onto plates and top with the tomato sauce and cashew mixture. Garnish with nutritional yeast (optional). Enjoy!

Ingredients

3/4 tsp Extra Virgin Olive Oil
8 ozs Extra Lean Ground Beef
1/4 tsp Sea Salt (divided)
3/4 cup Tomato Sauce
1/2 cup Cashews (soaked, drained, and rinsed)
1/4 Lemon (juiced)
3/4 tsp Nutritional Yeast
2 2/3 tbsps Water
1 Zucchini (medium, ends trimmed)

Notes

Storage
Refrigerate in an airtight container up to 2 days.

Vegetarian & Vegan
Use lentils instead of ground beef and adjust tomato sauce
as needed.

No Lemon
Use apple cider vinegar instead.

No Cashews
Use macadamia nuts instead.

Citrus Glazed Salmon

8 ingredients · 25 minutes · 2 servings

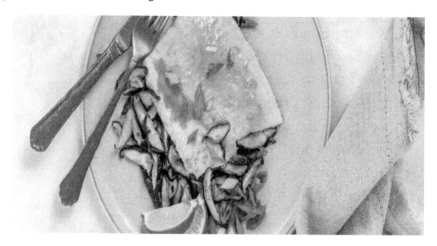

Directions

1. Preheat the oven to 350°F (177°C). Place the salmon in an oven-safe baking dish and drizzle with half of the extra virgin olive oil and season with half the sea salt. Bake for 13 to 16 minutes, until cooked through and flaky.

2. In a skillet over medium-high heat, add the remaining extra virgin olive oil. Add half of the green onions, mushrooms, and the remaining sea salt. Cook for 5 to 6 minutes, until the mushrooms and green onion are lightly browned and cooked through.

3. In a small bowl, whisk together the orange juice, coconut aminos, lime juice and zest.

4. Add the salmon to a platter along with the mushroom mixture and remaining raw green onions. Drizzle the sauce over top. Serve and enjoy!

Ingredients

8 ozs Salmon Fillet
1 tbsp Extra Virgin Olive Oil (divided)
1/4 tsp Sea Salt (divided)
5 stalks Green Onion (chopped, divided)
1 1/2 cups Shiitake Mushrooms (stems removed, sliced)
1 tbsp Orange Juice
1 1/2 tbsps Coconut Aminos or low sodium soy sauce
1 Lime (juiced, zested)

Notes

Leftovers
Refrigerate in an airtight container for up to two days.

Additional Toppings
Top with sesame seeds. Serve with rice, cauliflower rice, leafy greens, or roasted veggies.

Grilled Mediterranean Chicken Kabobs

10 ingredients · 30 minutes · 2 servings

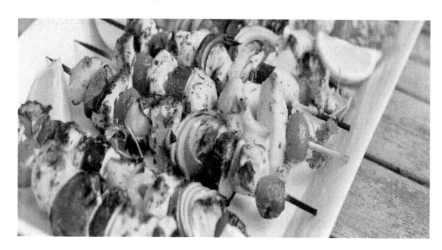

Directions

1. Combine the lemon juice, red wine vinegar, oregano and 1/2 of the olive oil in a mixing bowl. Add in the cubed chicken breast and mix well. Place in the fridge and let marinate while you prep the vegetables.

2. Dice the zucchini, yellow bell pepper, and red onion into large chunks. Toss in the remaining olive oil.

3. Slide the marinated cubed chicken, zucchini, yellow bell pepper, red onion, and cherry tomatoes onto the skewers.

4. Preheat the grill to medium heat and grill the kabobs for 8 to 10 minutes per side or until chicken is cooked through.

Ingredients
1/2 Lemon (juiced)
1 1/2 tsps Red Wine Vinegar
1 1/2 tsps Oregano (dried)
1 tbsp Extra Virgin Olive Oil (divided)
8 ozs Chicken Breast (boneless, skinless, diced into cubes)
1/2 Zucchini (large)
1/2 Yellow Bell Pepper
1/2 cup Red Onion
1 cup Cherry Tomatoes
4 Barbecue Skewers

Notes

Serving Size
One serving is equal to approximately two kabobs.

Serve Them With
Wild or brown rice, quinoa, grilled sweet potatoes and/or
tzatziki sauce. Add to leafy greens to make a salad.

Wooden Skewers
If grilling with wooden skewers, be sure to soak them in
water before using to avoid them catching fire on the grill.

Turkey Chili

14 ingredients · 40 minutes · 2 servings

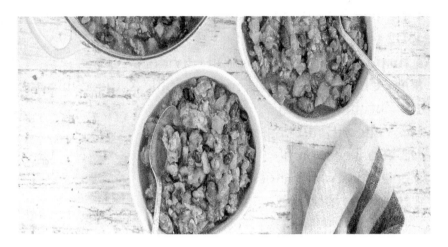

Directions

1. Heat oil in a large Dutch oven over medium heat. Add the ground turkey and onion and sauté for about five to seven minutes, or until the turkey is cooked through.

2. Add all of the remaining ingredients and stir to combine. Bring to a boil, then reduce the heat and simmer for 30 minutes.

3. Divide into bowls, serve, and enjoy!

Ingredients

3/4 tsp Extra Virgin Olive Oil
4 ozs Extra Lean Ground Turkey
1/4 Yellow Onion (chopped)

1/2 cup Diced Tomatoes
1/2 cup Crushed Tomatoes
1/2 cup Black Beans (cooked, rinsed)
1/2 cup Red Kidney Beans (cooked, rinsed)
1/2 Carrot (chopped)
1 1/4 stalks Celery (chopped)
1/4 Red Bell Pepper (chopped)
1/4 Jalapeno Pepper (chopped note use gloves)
2 1/4 tsps Chili Powder
1/4 tsp Cumin
1/4 tsp Sea Salt

Notes

Leftovers
Refrigerate in an airtight container for up to two days or freeze for up to two months.

Serving Size
One serving is equal to approximately two cups of chili.

More Veggies
Add sliced mushrooms, sliced kale, or baby spinach.

Ginger Chicken Bowl

9 ingredients · 20 minutes · 2 servings

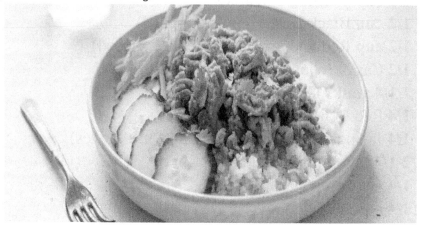

Directions

1. Heat a skillet over medium heat. Add half the oil and then the cauliflower rice. Sauté for five to seven minutes, then remove and set aside.

2. In the same pan, over medium-high heat, add the remaining oil and ground chicken and cook for five minutes, breaking apart into smaller pieces.

3. Add in coconut aminos, ginger, and garlic. Cook for another five minutes, until cooked through and golden.

4. Divide the cauliflower rice onto plates. Top with the ground chicken, cucumber, carrots, and cilantro. Enjoy!

Ingredients

1 tbsp Extra Virgin Olive Oil (divided)
3 cups Cauliflower Rice
1 lb Extra Lean Ground Chicken
2 tbsps Coconut Aminos
1 tsp Ground Ginger
1 tsp Garlic Powder
1/2 Cucumber (sliced)
1 Carrot (medium, peeled, and grated)
1/4 cup Cilantro (chopped)

Notes

Leftovers
Refrigerate in an airtight container for up to two days.

More Flavor
Use fresh ginger and garlic in place of ground ginger and garlic powder.

Additional Toppings
Swap cilantro out for mint for a fresh twist.

Spiced Cauliflower Rice Bowl

13 ingredients · 40 minutes · 1 serving

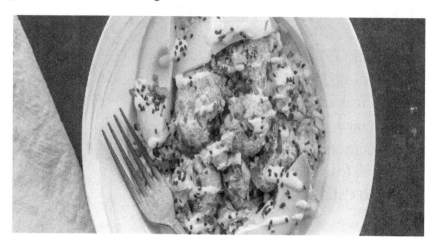

Directions

1. Preheat the oven to 400°F (204°C) and line a baking sheet with parchment paper.

2. Cook the brown rice according to the directions on the package. Once finished cooking, add the sea salt to the rice and mix.

3. While the rice cooks, add the cauliflower to a medium-sized bowl and toss with the turmeric, paprika and thyme. Place on the baking sheet and bake for 30 to 35 minutes.

4. In a small bowl whisk together the tahini, garlic, lemon juice and water. Set aside.

5. Divide the rice between bowls and top with cauliflower, avocado, cilantro, and sesame seeds. Drizzle the tahini dressing over top.

Ingredients

1/3 cup Brown Rice (dry, uncooked)
1/8 tsp Sea Salt
1/4 head Cauliflower (chopped into florets)
1/8 tsp Turmeric
1/4 tsp Paprika
1/4 tsp Thyme (dried)
1 tbsp Tahini
1/2 Garlic (clove, minced)
1 1/2 tsps Lemon Juice
1 1/2 tsps Water
1/2 Avocado (sliced)
2 tbsps Cilantro (chopped)
1/2 tsp Sesame Seeds (for topping)

Notes

Additional Toppings
Add protein to the dish such as baked tofu, chickpeas, or grilled chicken.

No Brown Rice
Use jasmine rice, cauliflower rice, quinoa, or millet instead.

Future Dietary Eating Plan

Now that you have followed a healthy diet for six weeks and removed sugar, gluten, dairy, and other inflammatory foods allowing you to transition from the Standard American Diet to a healthier lower carbohydrate diet; you need to decide which type of diet you wish to follow for the next thirty days.

I suggest thirty days because you may feel ready to try a more restrictive diet for a short period of time or not feel ready to commit to a dietary plan for long term. I have found that creating thirty, sixty and ninety day plans allow for a greater success rate than 'the rest of your life'. You decide what you feel comfortable with.

A low glycemic diet with intermittent fasting, and proper portion sizes (as explained earlier in the book) is helpful for many people; however some people need to drop their carbohydrate intake even further to promote weight loss and force their body to use more glucose from stored fat cells by creating ketones and following a Ketogenic Diet, There are pros and cons to each, and you may decide to follow a Keto Diet for thirty days and then re-evaluate.

A low carbohydrate diet keeps a higher amount of fibre, vitamins, minerals from fruits and vegetables in the diet. For people who suffer from constipation, this may be a better alternative. It may feel more comfortable to you as it is closer to the old diet you were following. A low carbohydrate diet is easier when travelling, in restaurants, and on special occasions for most people. However, there is also greater risk of sliding back into old eating habits and letting in a greater amount of old food favourites.

The Keto Diet has been shown in scientific studies to be effective in short term (30, 60, 90 day) and long term (up to 1 year) for creating fat loss, lower blood glucose and easier blood glucose balancing and reducing inflammation in the body. Now remember that I am not talking about the crazy Keto Diet you read about where people are eating high amounts of unhealthy fats and eating crazy things like butter in their coffee (yuck!) or massive amounts of high fat meats such as bacon or processed meats high in triglycerides and saturated fats, but the healthier version I outlined earlier in the book.

Whichever diet you choose to follow, create your meal plans, purchase the healthy foods you will be eating and track your meals using whichever online app you feel comfortable with. I recommend keeping a record of your food, your activity level, glucose levels, and how you feel so that you can show these results to your doctor and nutritionist. We all tend to forget what we have eaten, how much and how we felt, so tracking is very important.

When you have completed your thirty days (or whichever length of time you chose), set another goal to accomplish. Keep working on creating healthy habits and reminding yourself of your vision of a healthy body and life. Insulin resistance, and Type 2 diabetes can be reversed, and you are worthy of an amazing healthy life!

About the Author

Shawn Elliot is a Registered Holistic Nutritionist who specializes in weight loss and healing the body naturally through food and lifestyle. Her motto is "life is about balance not perfection" and encourages her clients to enjoy a piece of dark chocolate or occasional glass of wine.

After a fifteen year career in Human Resources, Shawn traded in her business suits and returned to school to pursue her love of nutrition and health. She is passionate about helping women take back control of their weight, their health, and their life. She has admitted to hating the cold and wet of Canadian winters and now travels between Canada and Mexico each year following the warmth of the sun. She loves the freedom of working online which allows her to work with women all over North America. When she isn't working with clients or writing, Shawn can be found puttering in her garden or curled up with a good book.

To learn more about nutrition and living a healthy life, go to www.powerfulevenutrition.com or contact Shawn at info@powerfulevenutrition.com

Made in the USA
Middletown, DE
08 December 2022

17416120R00219